LEAKY GUT

The Complete Guide to Fixing Leaky Gut and Supporting Women's Health

Dr. Amelia Grace Harper

Copyright © 2025 Dr. Amelia Grace Harper

All rights reserved.

ISBN: 9798304480543

CONTENTS

Introduction 7

Chapter 1: Understanding Leaky Gut:
What It Is and Why It Matters to Women 9

Chapter 2: The Science Behind Leaky Gut:
Why Your Body is Telling You Something 30

Chapter 3: The Key Causes of Leaky Gut in Women:
Hormones, Diet, and Lifestyle 48

Chapter 4: Leaky Gut and Women's Health Conditions:
The Hidden Link 72

Chapter 5: Nutrition for Healing Leaky Gut:
The Best Foods to Eat 95

Chapter 6: A 30-Day Leaky Gut Healing Plan for Women ...117

Chapter 7: Lifestyle Changes to Support
Long-Term Gut Health 141

Chapter 8: Beyond Leaky Gut:
Supporting Hormonal Balance and Overall Wellness 170

Chapter 9: Success Stories:
Real Women Who Healed Their Gut 190

Chapter 10: Frequently Asked Questions
About Leaky Gut and Women's Health 204

Conclusion 218

References 221

About the Author 224

Disclaimer: 226

Acknowledgments 229

Introduction

The Leaky Gut Epidemic—Why It Matters for Women's Health

Have you ever felt constantly fatigued, struggled with bloating or digestive issues, or experienced mood swings, skin problems, or hormonal imbalances that just don't seem to make sense? These symptoms are more than just annoyances—they could be signs of a much larger issue: **Leaky Gut Syndrome**. This condition, though not widely discussed, is becoming an increasingly common underlying cause of health challenges that particularly affect women.

Leaky gut, also known as intestinal permeability, occurs when the lining of the gut becomes damaged, allowing harmful substances like toxins, undigested food particles, and harmful bacteria to leak into the bloodstream. This triggers widespread inflammation and immune system responses that can lead to chronic illness and a host of symptoms that impact every part of your life. What many don't realize is that **leaky gut can be the hidden culprit behind everything from digestive problems to autoimmune conditions, hormonal imbalances, and even mental health struggles**.

For years, women have been suffering in silence, unsure of why they feel "off" or why common treatments don't seem to provide lasting relief. Whether it's the frustration of trying countless diets, medications, or supplements with little to no success, the impact of a leaky gut can be deeply discouraging. But here's the good news: **You don't have to accept living with these issues. There is a solution—and it starts with understanding the true cause of your symptoms and taking actionable steps to heal your body from the inside out.**

In this book, *Leaky Gut: The Complete Guide to Fixing Leaky Gut and Supporting Women's Health*, we will explore the science behind this condition, the unique ways it affects women, and most importantly, the steps you can take to heal your gut and transform your health. This book isn't just about fixing digestive problems; it's about empowering you to reclaim your energy, balance your hormones, heal your skin, and take control of your well-being.

We'll dive deep into the causes of leaky gut, from food sensitivities and hormonal imbalances to the stressors and environmental factors that contribute to its development. You'll learn how your gut health is directly linked to conditions like autoimmune diseases, chronic fatigue, and even mood disorders, many of which are more common in women.

But healing your gut doesn't stop with understanding the science. You'll also discover **practical, actionable steps to heal your gut** through diet, lifestyle changes, supplements, and stress management techniques—all tailored specifically to the needs of women. Whether you're dealing with PCOS, endometriosis, thyroid imbalances, or just general gut discomfort, this book will give you a roadmap to restore balance and support long-term health.

As you turn the pages, you'll find not only the latest scientific research but also **step-by-step guides, 30-day healing protocols, meal plans, and empowering success stories** from women who have healed their guts and transformed their lives. Whether you are just beginning your healing journey or looking for more effective ways to manage your leaky gut, this book will give you the knowledge and tools you need to feel your best—every single day.

It's time to take control of your health and start feeling like yourself again. **Let's heal your gut, restore balance to your body, and give you the freedom to live your life to the fullest.**

Welcome to the journey to better health—one step at a time.

Chapter 1: Understanding Leaky Gut: What It Is and Why It Matters to Women

Leaky gut syndrome is a condition that has gained attention in recent years, yet it remains misunderstood by many. If you've been experiencing persistent digestive issues, chronic fatigue, mood swings, skin breakouts, or unexplained pain, **leaky gut could be the underlying cause**, and it's especially relevant for women. Understanding this condition is the first step toward healing and restoring balance to your body. In this chapter, we'll define what leaky gut is, explore how it affects women, and delve into why it matters to your overall health.

What Is Leaky Gut Syndrome?

The human gut is lined with a layer of epithelial cells, which form tight junctions that regulate what passes through the digestive tract into the bloodstream. These tight junctions are crucial for maintaining gut barrier integrity, controlling the absorption of nutrients, and preventing harmful substances from entering the bloodstream. In a healthy gut, these tight junctions function properly, allowing nutrients to be absorbed while blocking harmful toxins, bacteria, and undigested food particles from passing through.

However, when the gut lining becomes damaged, these junctions loosen, causing gaps to form between the cells. As a result, **toxins,**

pathogens, and partially digested food particles leak into the bloodstream, leading to widespread inflammation and triggering an immune response. This is referred to as "intestinal permeability," or more commonly, **leaky gut**.

The consequences of leaky gut go far beyond digestive issues. It's linked to a variety of chronic health problems, including autoimmune diseases, food sensitivities, inflammation, and even mood disorders like anxiety and depression.

How Does Leaky Gut Affect Women?

While leaky gut can affect anyone, it's especially impactful for women due to the unique physiological and hormonal factors that influence their health. Here are several ways leaky gut specifically impacts women:

1. **Hormonal Imbalances**
   Women are particularly susceptible to hormonal imbalances, and these imbalances can worsen or even cause leaky gut. For example, **estrogen dominance**—a condition in which estrogen levels are too high relative to progesterone—can contribute to gut inflammation, disrupting the gut barrier and increasing intestinal permeability. Conditions like **PCOS (Polycystic Ovary Syndrome)** and **endometriosis** are also often linked to poor gut health, exacerbating both hormonal and digestive symptoms.

2. **Autoimmune Conditions**
   Women are far more likely to develop autoimmune diseases than men. **Autoimmune conditions** such as Hashimoto's thyroiditis, rheumatoid arthritis, and lupus are linked to leaky gut. In fact, the leaking of undigested food particles and toxins can trigger immune system responses that mistakenly attack healthy tissues in the body, leading to autoimmune flare-ups. When the immune system is compromised by a leaky gut, the body may begin to attack its own organs and tissues, leading to chronic inflammation and disease.

3. **Gut and Mental Health**
   The gut-brain connection is powerful, especially for women. Recent research has shown that the gut is often referred to as the

"second brain," as it contains millions of neurons and produces neurotransmitters like serotonin, which plays a major role in mood regulation. **Leaky gut** can disrupt this delicate balance, potentially leading to **mental health issues such as anxiety, depression, and brain fog**. Women are particularly vulnerable to these conditions, as hormonal fluctuations—especially during menstruation, pregnancy, and menopause—can amplify symptoms.

4. **Digestive Discomfort**

   Bloating, gas, constipation, and diarrhea are some of the most common digestive symptoms of leaky gut. Women are more likely to experience these symptoms due to hormonal fluctuations and changes in gut motility. Estrogen and progesterone, in particular, can slow down the digestive system, leading to uncomfortable bloating and irregular bowel movements. Additionally, women may also experience **food sensitivities** or intolerances that are linked to gut permeability, making it harder to enjoy a wide variety of foods without discomfort.

5. **Skin Issues**

   Skin problems like acne, eczema, rosacea, and psoriasis are often exacerbated by leaky gut. The connection between gut health and skin health is increasingly recognized in medical literature, with many skin conditions being considered "gut disorders in disguise." The chronic inflammation triggered by leaky gut can lead to **flare-ups of inflammatory skin conditions**, especially in women, who may experience skin problems linked to hormonal changes, stress, and diet.

Symptoms of Leaky Gut in Women

Recognizing the symptoms of leaky gut is crucial in diagnosing and addressing the condition. Since leaky gut impacts multiple systems in the body, the symptoms can vary widely. Some of the most common signs of leaky gut in women include:

- **Chronic digestive issues** (bloating, gas, diarrhea, or constipation)

- **Fatigue** and **brain fog**
- **Hormonal imbalances**, including PMS, heavy periods, or difficulty losing weight
- **Autoimmune flare-ups** or conditions like thyroid disorders
- **Skin problems**, including acne, eczema, or psoriasis
- **Frequent infections** or an impaired immune system
- **Mood swings**, anxiety, or depression
- **Food sensitivities** or intolerance to foods you once tolerated

If you've been dealing with any combination of these symptoms, it may be a sign that your gut is struggling to function properly. The good news is that healing leaky gut can address many of these issues at their root cause.

Why Leaky Gut Matters to Women's Health

Understanding and addressing leaky gut is essential for overall health, but for women, it is particularly transformative. The good news is that with the right tools, knowledge, and approach, **you can heal your gut** and restore balance to your digestive, hormonal, and immune systems. By focusing on healing the gut lining and reducing inflammation, women can experience profound improvements in their health—gaining energy, improving mental clarity, balancing hormones, and reducing the risk of chronic disease.

In the chapters ahead, you'll discover how to recognize the root causes of leaky gut, implement practical dietary and lifestyle changes, and follow a step-by-step healing protocol designed specifically for women. Whether you're looking to ease hormonal imbalances, clear up skin issues, or simply feel better in your body, healing your gut will be your ultimate tool for achieving lasting wellness.

Definition: Clear Explanation of "Leaky Gut" (Intestinal Permeability), Why It's Important, and How It Impacts Overall Health

Leaky gut syndrome, also known as **intestinal permeability**, is a condition where the lining of your small intestine becomes damaged, causing gaps to form between the cells that line the intestinal walls. This disruption allows harmful substances—such as undigested food particles, toxins, and harmful bacteria—to leak through these gaps and enter the bloodstream. The body's immune system then reacts to these foreign particles as though they are pathogens, triggering inflammation and potentially leading to a variety of chronic health issues.

To understand leaky gut, it's important to first understand the role of the gut in maintaining overall health. The gut, also known as the digestive tract, plays a crucial role in breaking down food, absorbing nutrients, and protecting the body from harmful substances. A healthy gut lining acts as a barrier that selectively allows nutrients to pass into the bloodstream while blocking toxins and harmful microorganisms from entering.

What Happens in Leaky Gut Syndrome?

The small intestine is lined with **intestinal epithelial cells** that are tightly bound together by structures known as **tight junctions**. These tight junctions regulate what passes between the cells into the bloodstream. Under normal circumstances, the gut lining is semi-permeable, meaning it only allows the passage of necessary nutrients and beneficial substances, such as amino acids, vitamins, and minerals, while preventing harmful particles like bacteria, toxins, and undigested food from entering the bloodstream.

In the case of **leaky gut**, the tight junctions begin to loosen, resulting in gaps or openings between the cells. These openings allow **large, undigested food particles**, **toxins**, and **pathogenic microbes** to escape from the intestines and enter the bloodstream. Once these substances enter the bloodstream, the body's immune system recognizes them as invaders and mounts an immune response, often leading to **chronic inflammation**.

This chronic inflammation can result in a range of health issues, because the immune system remains in a constant state of alert, attacking both harmful substances and sometimes even healthy tissues in the body. Over time, this can lead to the development of autoimmune diseases, food sensitivities, digestive disorders, skin conditions, and a variety of other health concerns.

Why Is Leaky Gut Important?

Leaky gut is important because it represents a breakdown of the body's ability to regulate what enters the bloodstream, which can have a cascading effect on multiple systems throughout the body. **The gut is** often referred to as the "second brain" because of the vital role it plays in managing not only digestion but also immune function, mental health, and overall well-being. When the integrity of the gut lining is compromised, it can disrupt the balance of these systems, leading to a wide array of symptoms and conditions.

Here are a few reasons why **leaky gut** is crucial to address:
1. **Immune System Overload**: The body's immune system is responsible for defending against harmful invaders, but when leaky gut occurs, the immune system becomes overburdened by the constant attack on foreign substances entering the bloodstream. This chronic immune activation can lead to **inflammation**, a common cause of many chronic diseases.
2. **Systemic Inflammation**: Chronic inflammation, which originates from leaky gut, is at the root of many diseases. **Inflammatory conditions** such as rheumatoid arthritis, cardiovascular disease, and even cancer have been linked to prolonged inflammation, much of which starts in the gut. Because the gut is where the immune system is closely connected to the body's overall health, when inflammation begins in the gut, it can easily spread throughout the body.
3. **Gut and Brain Communication**: The gut has an essential role in mental health through what is called the **gut-brain axis**—a two-way communication system that links the gut and the brain. **Leaky gut** can disrupt this communication, potentially leading to mental health issues such as anxiety, depression, and brain fog. Neurotransmitters like serotonin, which regulate mood, are primarily produced in the gut. When the gut is compromised, it can negatively affect mental clarity and emotional well-being.
4. **Hormonal Imbalances**: Leaky gut is also linked to **hormonal disruptions**. The gut is crucial for metabolizing and detoxifying hormones, and when it becomes leaky, it can interfere with the body's ability to regulate hormones like estrogen, progesterone, and cortisol. **Estrogen dominance** is one of the most common hormonal imbalances caused by a leaky gut, and this condition can lead to symptoms like heavy periods, weight gain, mood

swings, and even conditions like **polycystic ovary syndrome (PCOS)** and **endometriosis**.

5. **Autoimmune Diseases**: Leaky gut is strongly associated with the development of **autoimmune diseases**. The immune system can begin to attack the body's own tissues, mistakenly identifying them as harmful invaders. Conditions like **rheumatoid arthritis, Hashimoto's thyroiditis, lupus**, and **multiple sclerosis (MS)** have all been linked to leaky gut. When the intestinal barrier becomes compromised, it triggers an immune response that can attack the tissues of vital organs, leading to chronic and debilitating diseases.

6. **Nutrient Deficiency**: The breakdown of the gut lining can also result in **malabsorption** of essential nutrients. Even if you're eating a balanced diet, leaky gut can prevent your body from properly absorbing vital nutrients like vitamins, minerals, and amino acids. This can lead to deficiencies that exacerbate other health problems, contributing to symptoms such as fatigue, weakened immunity, and poor skin health.

7. **Increased Food Sensitivities**: Leaky gut is often accompanied by food intolerances or sensitivities. Because the immune system is hyper-reactive due to the leakage of undigested food particles into the bloodstream, it may begin to overreact to certain foods, especially those that are more difficult to digest, like gluten, dairy, or refined sugars. **Food sensitivities** often manifest as digestive discomfort, skin rashes, headaches, or joint pain.

How Leaky Gut Impacts Overall Health

Leaky gut is not just a digestive issue; it is a **systemic problem** that affects nearly every aspect of your health. Here's how it can disrupt various areas of your life:

- **Digestive Health**: The most immediate and noticeable impact of leaky gut is on digestion. You may experience bloating, gas, diarrhea, constipation, or even irritable bowel syndrome (IBS). The gut lining is directly responsible for absorbing nutrients and filtering out waste, so when it becomes permeable, digestion suffers.

- **Immune System Health**: A compromised gut lining is often the precursor to an immune system that is constantly on high alert. This leads to **chronic inflammation**, which can cause a host of health problems ranging from joint pain to cardiovascular disease. The immune system's constant activation is a primary cause of conditions like autoimmune diseases.
- **Mental Health**: Since so many of the neurotransmitters responsible for regulating mood are produced in the gut, leaky gut can have a profound effect on **mental clarity, memory**, and **emotional stability**. Anxiety, depression, and brain fog are common consequences of an unhealthy gut-brain connection.
- **Skin Health**: Leaky gut is also a common underlying cause of **skin conditions** such as acne, eczema, and psoriasis. The inflammation triggered by leaky gut can cause flare-ups, leading to irritated, red, or inflamed skin. **Gut health and skin health** are intimately connected, which is why healing the gut often leads to clearer skin.
- **Weight Management**: Leaky gut can contribute to **weight gain** and difficulty losing weight due to its impact on hormones like insulin, cortisol, and leptin, which regulate hunger, metabolism, and fat storage. Balancing the gut can be a powerful tool for restoring a healthy weight.

Definition: Clear Explanation of "Leaky Gut" (Intestinal Permeability), Why It's Important, and How It Impacts Overall Health

Leaky gut syndrome, also known as **intestinal permeability**, is a condition where the lining of your intestines becomes damaged, leading to gaps or openings between the epithelial cells that form the walls of the gut. These cells, under normal circumstances, are tightly joined together by structures called **tight junctions**, which act as a barrier to control what passes from the intestines into the bloodstream. When these junctions weaken or become compromised, larger-than-normal particles—including undigested food, toxins, bacteria, and waste—leak into the bloodstream, triggering an immune response and inflammation throughout the body. This process leads to a wide range of symptoms and can disrupt multiple systems in the body.

How the Gut Works Under Normal Conditions

The gut, also known as the digestive system, plays a critical role in both digestion and overall health. It serves as the body's first line of defense against harmful microorganisms and plays an essential part in nutrient absorption. The **intestinal lining** acts as a selective barrier, allowing only specific nutrients, such as amino acids, glucose, vitamins, and minerals, to pass through into the bloodstream. At the same time, it keeps out harmful substances, including pathogens, toxins, and large undigested food particles.

The intestinal lining is made up of **intestinal epithelial cells**. These cells are tightly bound together by **tight junctions**, which regulate what can and cannot pass through. This selective permeability ensures that essential nutrients are absorbed into the body while harmful substances are kept at bay. However, in **leaky gut syndrome**, the integrity of this barrier is compromised, leading to **intestinal hyperpermeability**.

What Happens in Leaky Gut Syndrome?

In a healthy digestive system, the gut lining forms a strong barrier that controls the passage of substances. However, when **leaky gut** occurs, these tight junctions loosen or break apart. This creates **gaps** or **holes** between the epithelial cells, which allows particles that should not normally pass through the lining—such as **undigested food particles**, **toxins**, and **bacteria**—to leak into the bloodstream.

Once these foreign particles enter the bloodstream, the body's immune system detects them as harmful invaders. In response, the immune system triggers an inflammatory response, which can lead to a wide range of problems. **Chronic inflammation** can have a cascade effect on the body, affecting everything from digestion to mental health to skin appearance.

Why Is Leaky Gut Important?

Leaky gut is important because it is not just a localized problem affecting the digestive tract—it can have far-reaching consequences on many aspects of health. When the gut becomes more permeable, harmful substances can enter the bloodstream, triggering immune system activation. This can result in chronic inflammation, autoimmune responses, and nutrient deficiencies that impact several bodily systems. Here are a few key reasons why leaky gut is critical to overall health:

1. **Chronic Inflammation**
   One of the most concerning outcomes of leaky gut is **chronic inflammation**. The immune system constantly responds to the leaked particles, leading to ongoing inflammation throughout the body. This is a major contributor to a wide array of health problems, including autoimmune conditions, cardiovascular disease, and even some cancers. Chronic inflammation can also affect the brain, leading to mental health issues like anxiety and depression.

2. **Immune System Dysfunction**
   The gut is home to about 70% of the body's immune cells. It is responsible for regulating immune responses and defending against harmful substances. When the gut barrier becomes compromised, the immune system becomes overstimulated, potentially leading to **autoimmune diseases**. Conditions such as rheumatoid arthritis, Hashimoto's thyroiditis, and lupus have all been associated with leaky gut syndrome. The immune system may also begin attacking the body's own tissues, a phenomenon known as **autoimmunity**.

3. **Nutrient Malabsorption**
   When the gut lining is damaged, it can interfere with the body's ability to properly absorb nutrients. Even if you're consuming a nutrient-rich diet, leaky gut may prevent the absorption of vitamins, minerals, and other essential nutrients. This can lead to **nutrient deficiencies**, which in turn may result in symptoms like fatigue, weakness, poor skin health, and impaired immune function. **Vitamin D, B vitamins, magnesium, and zinc** are just a few of the nutrients often impacted by a compromised gut.

4. **Mental Health Problems**
   The gut and brain are intimately connected through what is known as the **gut-brain axis**. This communication system links the digestive system and the central nervous system, allowing for the transfer of signals between the two. **Neurotransmitters** like

serotonin, which are produced in the gut, play a crucial role in regulating mood and behavior. When the gut lining is damaged, it can disrupt the production and function of these neurotransmitters, leading to mood swings, anxiety, depression, and even cognitive issues like brain fog.

5. **Hormonal Imbalances**

   Hormones are key regulators of many bodily functions, including metabolism, mood, and reproductive health. Leaky gut can interfere with the body's ability to regulate hormones properly. For example, **estrogen dominance**, a condition in which the body has too much estrogen relative to progesterone, is often linked to gut health issues. Hormonal imbalances caused by leaky gut can result in **PMS, heavy periods**, weight gain, and conditions like **polycystic ovary syndrome (PCOS)** and **endometriosis**.

6. **Skin Conditions**

   The health of your skin is closely connected to the health of your gut. **Leaky gut** has been associated with a variety of skin problems, such as **eczema, psoriasis**, acne, and rosacea. Chronic inflammation caused by the leakage of toxins into the bloodstream can trigger skin flare-ups and exacerbate existing conditions. Additionally, the gut microbiome (the community of bacteria in the gut) plays a major role in skin health, and an imbalance in gut bacteria can lead to skin issues.

7. **Food Sensitivities and Allergies**

   Leaky gut is often the underlying cause of **food sensitivities** and **food allergies**. When undigested food particles leak into the bloodstream, they can trigger an immune response that results in food sensitivities or intolerances. For example, people with leaky gut may develop an intolerance to gluten or dairy, even if they didn't have issues with these foods in the past. Over time, these sensitivities can contribute to more severe digestive and immune problems.

How Leaky Gut Impacts Overall Health

The impact of leaky gut extends far beyond the digestive system.

Here's a breakdown of how a compromised gut lining can affect your overall health:
- **Digestive Health**: The gut is the body's primary site of digestion and nutrient absorption. When the integrity of the gut lining is compromised, it leads to digestive issues such as bloating, gas, diarrhea, constipation, and irritable bowel syndrome (IBS). The gut's ability to process food and absorb nutrients is significantly impaired, leading to discomfort and malabsorption of nutrients.
- **Immune Health**: The gut is the largest immune organ in the body, and leaky gut compromises its ability to defend against harmful microorganisms. Chronic exposure to bacteria and toxins in the bloodstream can overwhelm the immune system, contributing to the development of autoimmune conditions and systemic inflammation.
- **Mental Health**: With the gut-brain axis disrupted, leaky gut can lead to mood disorders such as anxiety, depression, and irritability. Cognitive issues like memory problems and brain fog can also result from the gut's inability to produce and regulate neurotransmitters like serotonin.
- **Hormonal Health**: Leaky gut interferes with the body's ability to metabolize and detoxify hormones, leading to imbalances. These imbalances can manifest in conditions like PMS, difficulty losing weight, and disorders such as PCOS and endometriosis.
- **Skin Health**: Since the gut plays a role in detoxification and immune regulation, leaky gut can contribute to skin issues like acne, eczema, and rosacea. The inflammation caused by leaky gut can trigger flare-ups of these conditions, making it harder to achieve clear, healthy skin.

Symptoms of Leaky Gut: Physical, Emotional, and Hormonal Symptoms Specific to Women

Leaky gut syndrome, also known as **intestinal permeability**, affects the body in profound ways, contributing to a variety of symptoms that impact a woman's **physical health, emotional well-being**, and **hormonal balance**. While the symptoms of leaky gut can vary from person to person, certain signs are commonly reported. Many of these symptoms are subtle and can easily be attributed to other conditions, making leaky gut a difficult diagnosis to pinpoint. However, understanding these symptoms, especially as they relate to women's health, can offer a crucial starting point for identifying and addressing this condition.

Physical Symptoms of Leaky Gut

1. **Bloating and Gas**
   One of the most common signs of leaky gut is **bloating**. The inflammation and imbalances caused by the leakage of toxins and undigested food particles into the bloodstream can disrupt the digestive process. This leads to discomfort, distension, and frequent **gas**. For women, bloating may also be cyclical, exacerbated around their menstrual cycle due to hormonal fluctuations that impact gut health.
   - **What You Might Feel**: A feeling of fullness or tightness in the stomach, visible swelling, or gas after eating certain foods—especially those high in fiber or that are difficult to digest, like beans, dairy, or cruciferous vegetables.

2. **Fatigue and Low Energy**
   Chronic **fatigue** is a frequent complaint for women dealing with leaky gut. The body's immune system is constantly activated due to the presence of toxins and harmful particles in the bloodstream. This constant state of **inflammation** can be draining and may leave women feeling chronically tired or exhausted, even after a full night's sleep. Additionally, leaky gut can interfere with nutrient absorption, leading to deficiencies in essential vitamins and minerals like **B vitamins**, **iron**, and **magnesium**, which are vital for energy production.
   - **What You Might Feel**: Persistent tiredness, difficulty getting out of bed in the morning, feeling fatigued throughout the day, and a general sense of low energy despite adequate sleep or rest.

3. **Brain Fog and Difficulty Concentrating**
   Brain fog is a common symptom associated with leaky gut, and it can significantly impair a woman's ability to focus, think clearly,

and remember things. This cognitive dysfunction is often linked to **chronic inflammation** in the body and the gut's inability to produce or regulate important neurotransmitters, like **serotonin** and **dopamine**, that influence mood, focus, and mental clarity. In some cases, the inflammation caused by leaky gut may even disrupt the gut-brain axis, further compounding mental fog and cognitive issues.

- **What You Might Feel**: Difficulty focusing, forgetfulness, mental sluggishness, trouble completing tasks, or feeling "spaced out" or disconnected.

4. **Digestive Issues (Diarrhea and Constipation)**
Women with leaky gut may experience a range of **digestive issues**, including **diarrhea, constipation**, or alternating between the two. The disruption of the gut lining can interfere with normal bowel movements, causing irregularity in the digestive process. For some, the presence of undigested food particles in the bloodstream can further upset the digestive tract, causing irritation and **gut dysbiosis** (imbalance in gut bacteria).

- **What You Might Feel**: Frequent trips to the bathroom with either very loose stools or difficulty passing stool, abdominal cramping, or a feeling of incomplete bowel movements.

5. **Food Sensitivities and Allergies**
A damaged intestinal lining can lead to the development of **food sensitivities** and **food allergies** that were not present before. This is because the leakage of undigested food particles into the bloodstream can trigger an **immune response**, causing the body to mistakenly identify certain foods as harmful. Women with leaky gut may develop sensitivities to common foods like **gluten**, **dairy**, or **soy**, and experience reactions ranging from digestive upset to skin rashes or migraines.

- **What You Might Feel**: Gassiness, bloating, or nausea after eating certain foods; unexplained headaches; skin rashes; or symptoms of **eczema** or **hives**.

Emotional Symptoms of Leaky Gut

1. **Mood Swings**
   Women with leaky gut often experience **mood swings** that are tied to both the chronic inflammation in the body and the disruption of the **gut-brain axis**. Since the gut plays an essential role in the production of neurotransmitters like **serotonin** (often called the "happy hormone"), damage to the gut lining can lead to imbalances in mood-regulating chemicals. Additionally, the constant activation of the immune system can make women feel irritable, anxious, or depressed, even without a clear emotional trigger.
   - **What You Might Feel**: Sudden shifts in mood, feeling overly emotional, getting frustrated or upset easily, or experiencing periods of sadness or irritability without a clear cause.
2. **Anxiety and Depression**
   Chronic **anxiety** and **depression** are frequently reported in women with leaky gut. The gut and brain are intimately connected, and a disrupted gut microbiome can alter the production of important neurotransmitters that regulate mood, such as **serotonin** and **dopamine**. The chronic inflammation associated with leaky gut also activates the body's **stress response**, leading to feelings of unease, anxiety, and persistent sadness.
   - **What You Might Feel**: General anxiety, panic attacks, persistent feelings of sadness or hopelessness, or a lack of motivation to do everyday activities.
3. **Irritability**
   Leaky gut can contribute to **irritability** and a feeling of being easily agitated. The constant state of inflammation in the body and the gut's inability to absorb nutrients properly can leave women feeling mentally and emotionally worn out. Stress, anxiety, and poor sleep, which often accompany leaky gut, can further exacerbate irritability.
   - **What You Might Feel**: Frustration over small things, snapping at others, or feeling impatient even when there

is no obvious reason for the irritation.

Hormonal Symptoms Specific to Women

1. **Irregular Periods and PMS**
Hormonal imbalances are a hallmark of leaky gut, especially for women. The **gut microbiome** plays a significant role in regulating estrogen metabolism, and when leaky gut disrupts this balance, women may experience **irregular menstrual cycles** or **increased PMS** symptoms. These imbalances can manifest as heavy periods, spotting between cycles, or skipped periods. Leaky gut may also worsen **PMS symptoms**, including mood swings, cramps, and fatigue.
    - **What You Might Feel**: Changes in cycle length, increased pain or cramping, heavier or lighter flow, and mood swings around your period.

2. **Estrogen Dominance**
Estrogen dominance occurs when there is too much estrogen relative to other hormones like **progesterone**. This imbalance can lead to a range of symptoms, including **irregular periods**, **fibroids, endometriosis**, or **PCOS** (polycystic ovary syndrome). Leaky gut interferes with the body's ability to detoxify and excrete excess estrogen properly, exacerbating this imbalance.
    - **What You Might Feel**: Bloating, tender breasts, heavy or irregular periods, or increased symptoms of endometriosis or fibroids.

3. **Weight Gain and Difficulty Losing Weight**
Hormonal disruptions caused by leaky gut can also lead to weight gain, especially around the **abdomen**. Leaky gut is linked to increased **insulin resistance** and changes in **metabolism**, making it harder for women to lose weight. Chronic inflammation may also cause the body to retain water or store fat more easily. Women may find that despite efforts to eat healthily or exercise, they struggle to maintain or lose weight.
    - **What You Might Feel**: Inability to lose weight, unexplained weight gain, or changes in body composition, especially around the belly.

4. **Thyroid Issues**

Leaky gut can contribute to **autoimmune thyroid conditions**, such as **Hashimoto's thyroiditis**, due to the disruption of the immune system. Chronic inflammation and immune system activation increase the likelihood of the body mistakenly attacking its own tissues, including the thyroid gland. Thyroid dysfunction can result in **fatigue, hair loss, weight gain, cold intolerance**, and other symptoms.

- **What You Might Feel**: Dry skin, thinning hair, cold hands or feet, fatigue, and weight gain despite no significant change in diet or exercise.

How Leaky Gut Relates to Hormonal Imbalances: Understanding the Gut-Hormone Connection in Women

The **gut-hormone connection** is one of the most important yet often overlooked aspects of health, particularly for women who experience a range of hormonal imbalances. **Leaky gut syndrome**, or **intestinal permeability**, has been increasingly recognized as a potential contributor to a variety of hormonal disturbances. For women, this connection is especially crucial because the gut plays a vital role in regulating the balance of key hormones like **estrogen, progesterone**, and **cortisol**. When the gut becomes compromised, it can lead to a cascade of hormonal disruptions that affect everything from the menstrual cycle to stress management and even weight gain. Understanding how leaky gut impacts these hormones is key to addressing the root cause of many chronic health conditions that women face.

The Gut-Hormone Connection: A Brief Overview

The gut is not just the body's digestive system; it is a complex network of **microorganisms** (gut microbiota) that influences almost every aspect of health, including hormone production, metabolism, and immune function. In a healthy gut, nutrients are absorbed efficiently, the immune system is well-regulated, and the intestinal lining serves as a protective barrier to prevent harmful substances from entering the bloodstream.

In cases of leaky gut, the intestinal lining becomes damaged and porous. This allows **toxins, undigested food particles**, and **pathogens** to leak into the bloodstream, which can trigger widespread inflammation and immune activation. This chronic inflammation disrupts the normal functioning of the **endocrine system** (the system responsible for hormone production), leading to **hormonal imbalances** that can affect various bodily functions. For women, the most notable imbalances occur in **estrogen, progesterone,** and **cortisol**—key hormones that regulate everything from the menstrual cycle to mood and metabolism.

Leaky Gut and Estrogen Imbalance

Estrogen is a **primary sex hormone** that plays a central role in the **menstrual cycle, fertility,** and **reproductive health**. In women, estrogen also influences the health of bones, the cardiovascular system, and even brain function. **Estrogen dominance**, a condition in which there is too much estrogen in relation to progesterone, is a common hormonal imbalance associated with leaky gut. Here's how leaky gut can contribute to estrogen issues:

1. **Impaired Estrogen Detoxification**
   One of the key functions of the **liver** is to process and **detoxify excess estrogen** through a process known as **estrogen metabolism**. A healthy gut microbiome plays a role in this by regulating enzymes that aid in the breakdown and elimination of estrogen. When the gut is damaged by leaky gut syndrome, it can alter the composition of the microbiome, leading to a disruption in estrogen detoxification. This can result in the **reabsorption of excess estrogen** back into the bloodstream, contributing to **estrogen dominance**.
   - **Symptoms of Estrogen Dominance**: Bloating, irregular periods, heavy menstrual flow, breast tenderness, mood swings, and headaches.

2. **Inflammation and Estrogen Receptors**
   Chronic **inflammation** caused by leaky gut may increase the body's sensitivity to estrogen. This means that estrogen receptors in tissues such as the **breasts, uterus,** and **ovaries** may become overstimulated, leading to the development of conditions like **fibroids, endometriosis,** or **breast tenderness**. Inflammation can also interfere with the proper signaling of estrogen, further

contributing to imbalances.
3. **Gut Dysbiosis and Estrogen**
An imbalance in gut bacteria (known as **dysbiosis**) can impact estrogen metabolism, as certain types of gut bacteria are responsible for the **metabolism of estrogens**. When these beneficial bacteria are depleted due to an unhealthy gut, the body's ability to properly break down and eliminate estrogen is compromised, leading to higher levels of circulating estrogen.

Leaky Gut and Progesterone Deficiency

Progesterone is another key **sex hormone** that plays a vital role in **regulating the menstrual cycle, supporting pregnancy,** and balancing the effects of estrogen. **Progesterone deficiency** often occurs in women with leaky gut, contributing to a number of hormonal issues. Here's how leaky gut may influence progesterone levels:

1. **Increased Cortisol Production**
Leaky gut leads to **systemic inflammation** and an overactive immune response. This constant state of **stress** can result in higher levels of **cortisol**, the body's primary stress hormone. Elevated cortisol levels can suppress the production of **progesterone** because the body prioritizes the production of cortisol during times of stress. This imbalance between estrogen and progesterone is a common cause of **PMS** and other menstrual irregularities.

2. **Immune Activation and Hormonal Disruption**
The constant activation of the immune system due to the presence of toxins and undigested food particles in the bloodstream can also interfere with **progesterone production**. In some cases, this can lead to **low progesterone levels**, which is a key factor in **estrogen dominance**. This imbalance is especially problematic for women who are trying to conceive or are struggling with infertility.
    - **Symptoms of Progesterone Deficiency**: Irregular periods, heavy or painful menstrual flow, trouble sleeping, anxiety, and difficulty getting pregnant.

3. **Poor Gut Function and Nutrient Deficiency**

Leaky gut can impair nutrient absorption, leading to **deficiencies** in vitamins and minerals that are essential for hormone production, including **magnesium, zinc**, and **vitamin B6**. These nutrients are critical for the production of progesterone, and a lack of them can contribute to **progesterone insufficiency**.

Leaky Gut and Cortisol Imbalance

Cortisol, often referred to as the **"stress hormone"**, plays a crucial role in regulating the body's response to stress. However, chronic stress and inflammation, like those caused by leaky gut, can lead to **chronic cortisol dysregulation**. Here's how leaky gut can contribute to **cortisol imbalances**:

1. **Inflammation and Cortisol Production**
   When the gut is compromised, it results in increased inflammation and immune activation. This activates the **hypothalamic-pituitary-adrenal (HPA) axis**, a system responsible for regulating the body's stress response. The HPA axis signals the **adrenal glands** to release cortisol. Chronic activation of this system, caused by leaky gut, can lead to **elevated cortisol levels**, which can further disrupt hormonal balance.

2. **Cortisol and Progesterone Suppression**
   Chronic stress and high cortisol levels can suppress **progesterone** production, further exacerbating the effects of **estrogen dominance** and contributing to **PMS** symptoms, **irregular cycles**, and other hormonal imbalances. High cortisol levels can also lead to **adrenal fatigue**, which affects the body's ability to respond to stress and can result in symptoms such as fatigue, weight gain, and difficulty sleeping.
   - **Symptoms of High Cortisol Levels**: Weight gain (especially around the belly), anxiety, difficulty sleeping, fatigue, and irritability.

The Gut-Hormone Axis: A Vital Feedback Loop

The **gut-hormone axis** operates in a feedback loop, where the health of the gut microbiome directly influences hormonal regulation, and vice versa. When the gut is inflamed due to leaky gut, this alters not only hormone production but also the ability of the body to detoxify and metabolize hormones properly. This creates a **vicious cycle** where hormonal imbalances feed into further gut dysfunction, leading to a variety of chronic health problems.

Chapter 2: The Science Behind Leaky Gut: Why Your Body is Telling You Something

Leaky gut, or **intestinal permeability**, is more than just a buzzword in the world of health and wellness—it's a profound condition that can trigger a cascade of issues throughout your body. While the concept of "leaky gut" has gained considerable attention in recent years, many are still uncertain about what it truly is and why it matters. This chapter will break down the science behind leaky gut, explain its underlying mechanisms, and explore why your body is trying to tell you something important when it signals that this condition is present. Understanding the physiological and biochemical processes behind leaky gut can help empower you to take steps toward healing.

What is Leaky Gut?

Leaky gut syndrome refers to an increase in **intestinal permeability**, where the lining of the small intestine becomes damaged, causing gaps to form between the cells of the intestinal walls. The **intestinal lining** serves as a protective barrier, allowing nutrients and water to pass through while preventing harmful substances like **toxins, undigested food particles**, and **pathogens** from entering the bloodstream.

When the gut lining is compromised, these harmful substances "leak" through the gaps into the bloodstream. This sets off a chain reaction of **immune system activation, inflammation**, and **immune responses**, which can lead to a variety of chronic health conditions. Leaky gut isn't just a localized digestive issue; it affects your entire body, from your gut microbiome to your brain, and from your skin to your hormones.

How the Intestinal Barrier Works: A Complex System

To understand leaky gut, it's essential to first grasp the role of the **intestinal barrier** and how it works under normal circumstances. The small intestine is lined with **intestinal epithelial cells**, which are tightly connected by structures called **tight junctions**. These junctions act like the seals of a door, controlling what enters and exits the bloodstream. Under normal conditions, these tight junctions allow only beneficial nutrients and small molecules to pass through into the bloodstream, while blocking larger molecules, such as bacteria, undigested food particles, and toxins, from getting through.

However, various factors can damage the integrity of the gut lining and loosen these tight junctions, leading to the condition known as **intestinal permeability** or leaky gut.

What Causes Leaky Gut?

Several factors contribute to the development of leaky gut, including lifestyle choices, environmental influences, and underlying health conditions. Some of the most significant contributors are:

1. Chronic Inflammation

Chronic inflammation, often caused by poor diet, stress, or environmental toxins, plays a central role in the development of leaky gut. **Inflammatory cytokines**, such as **TNF-alpha** (tumor necrosis factor-alpha) and **IL-6** (interleukin-6), are produced by immune cells in response to injury, infection, or irritants. These cytokines can damage the **tight junctions** between intestinal cells, causing them to weaken and separate, creating gaps through which harmful substances can leak into the bloodstream.

2. Poor Diet: High Sugar, Processed Foods, and Gluten

The foods you eat significantly influence the integrity of your gut lining. Diets high in **refined sugars, processed foods**, and **trans fats** have been shown to promote inflammation and damage the gut lining.

For instance, **gluten**—a protein found in wheat and other grains—can directly increase intestinal permeability, especially in those with **non-celiac gluten sensitivity**. Studies have shown that gluten can activate an immune response that damages the tight junctions in the small intestine, making it easier for harmful particles to enter the bloodstream.

3. Dysbiosis: Imbalance in Gut Microbiota

The gut is home to trillions of microorganisms, collectively known as the **gut microbiota**. A healthy and diverse microbiome supports the integrity of the intestinal barrier. However, **dysbiosis**—an imbalance in the gut microbiota—can lead to overgrowth of harmful bacteria and yeast, which can damage the gut lining and increase intestinal permeability. The gut microbiota plays a crucial role in regulating immune responses and inflammation, so an imbalance in these microbes can create a vicious cycle of chronic inflammation and leaky gut.

4. Stress and Cortisol

Chronic stress, both emotional and physical, can have a profound impact on gut health. When you are stressed, your body produces more of the **stress hormone cortisol**, which in high amounts can disrupt the function of the gut barrier. Cortisol suppresses the production of **beneficial gut bacteria**, alters gut motility, and reduces blood flow to the gut, leading to weakened intestinal cells. The combination of elevated cortisol levels and increased inflammation due to stress significantly contributes to the development of leaky gut.

5. Medications and Antibiotics

Certain medications, particularly **non-steroidal anti-inflammatory drugs (NSAIDs)**, antibiotics, and **proton pump inhibitors (PPIs)**, can damage the gut lining. **NSAIDs**, such as ibuprofen and aspirin, reduce the production of protective mucus in the stomach and intestines, leading to inflammation and potential leaky gut. Long-term use of **antibiotics** can disrupt the delicate balance of gut bacteria, reducing the diversity of beneficial microbes and promoting overgrowth of harmful bacteria. Similarly, **PPIs**, which are commonly used to treat acid reflux, can decrease the acidity in the stomach, impairing digestion and potentially allowing harmful pathogens to thrive in the intestines.

6. Food Sensitivities and Allergies

Food sensitivities, particularly to foods like **dairy, gluten, soy**, and **eggs**, can trigger immune responses that damage the intestinal lining. In some cases, these food triggers can cause an immune reaction called **leaky gut inflammation**, further exacerbating the condition. The body's immune system mistakenly identifies certain foods as threats, causing the release of inflammatory substances that break down the protective lining of the gut.

7. Environmental Toxins

Environmental pollutants, including **pesticides, heavy metals**, and **microplastics**, have also been shown to contribute to leaky gut. These toxins can irritate the gut lining and alter the gut microbiome, making it more susceptible to permeability. Furthermore, the body's inability to detoxify these harmful substances efficiently, due to the compromised gut barrier, can lead to systemic inflammation and a cascade of health problems.

The Role of Inflammation in Leaky Gut

The primary issue with leaky gut is the **inflammation** that it triggers throughout the body. When harmful substances enter the bloodstream, the immune system recognizes them as invaders and activates an immune response. This leads to the production of **inflammatory cytokines** and **antibodies** that circulate through the bloodstream, contributing to chronic inflammation in various tissues and organs. This systemic inflammation is at the root of many diseases, including autoimmune disorders, **irritable bowel syndrome (IBS), chronic fatigue syndrome, hormonal imbalances**, and **skin conditions** like eczema and acne.

How Leaky Gut Affects Overall Health

When the intestinal barrier becomes compromised, the implications go beyond digestive issues. The **immune system**, which is largely housed in the gut, becomes dysregulated. The gut microbiome, which plays a vital role in maintaining the immune system, becomes imbalanced, and this leads to **immune system dysfunction**. As a result, the body becomes more susceptible to chronic conditions such as:

- **Autoimmune Diseases**: Conditions like **rheumatoid arthritis, Hashimoto's thyroiditis**, and **lupus** can be triggered by the

immune system attacking the body's own tissues after leaky gut allows **autoantibodies** to circulate.
- **Skin Conditions**: **Acne, eczema,** and **psoriasis** are often linked to leaky gut, as systemic inflammation from the gut can manifest on the skin.
- **Mental Health Issues**: The gut-brain axis connects the gut microbiome to brain function. Leaky gut has been implicated in mood disorders like **anxiety, depression,** and **brain fog**.
- **Weight Gain and Metabolic Issues**: Chronic inflammation and hormonal imbalances caused by leaky gut can lead to **insulin resistance, weight gain,** and an increased risk of **metabolic syndrome**.

Why Your Body is Telling You Something Important

Leaky gut is a symptom of **systemic dysfunction** rather than a standalone condition. When your body signals that something is wrong—whether through digestive issues like bloating and gas, skin flare-ups, or mood swings—it's trying to alert you to the root cause: **intestinal permeability**. This dysfunction is often the body's way of signaling that the gut is under stress, that there is an imbalance in the microbiome, or that an autoimmune reaction is occurring. Addressing leaky gut is not just about treating symptoms; it's about understanding the bigger picture of **holistic health** and getting to the heart of systemic inflammation, gut health, and immune function.

Gut Health and Immunity: An In-Depth Look at How the Gut Impacts the Immune System and Autoimmune Diseases More Common in Women

The gut is often referred to as the body's "second brain" because of its powerful influence on our health. But more than just managing digestion, the **gut** also plays a pivotal role in regulating the **immune system**. In fact, approximately **70% of the body's immune system** resides in the **gut-associated lymphoid tissue** (GALT), making the health of the gut intrinsically linked to the overall function of the immune system. When the gut becomes unbalanced, it can lead to a cascade of immune system dysfunction, triggering conditions like **autoimmune diseases**, which are notably more common in women.

In this chapter, we will explore the intimate connection between gut health and immunity, shedding light on how an imbalance in the gut can not only impair your immune system but also contribute to the development of autoimmune conditions. Additionally, we will discuss why women are more susceptible to certain autoimmune diseases and how leaky gut and immune dysregulation might be contributing factors.

The Gut-Immune Connection: How It Works

The gut is home to a **vast network** of **immune cells**, and it serves as the first line of defense against harmful invaders like bacteria, viruses, and toxins. The **gut microbiome**, which refers to the trillions of bacteria, viruses, fungi, and other microorganisms that live in your digestive tract, plays an integral role in maintaining immune function.

1. Gut Microbiome and Immune Regulation

A healthy gut microbiome promotes the production of **anti-inflammatory cytokines** and supports the activity of **T-cells** and other immune cells that help defend against infections. Beneficial bacteria also help **train the immune system**, teaching it to differentiate between harmful invaders and harmless substances like food proteins and beneficial gut bacteria.

However, when the gut microbiome becomes **imbalanced** (a condition known as **dysbiosis**), harmful bacteria and other pathogens can proliferate, triggering an immune response. This chronic immune activation can lead to **systemic inflammation**, which is the precursor to many immune-related disorders, including autoimmune diseases.

2. Intestinal Permeability (Leaky Gut) and Immune Dysfunction

When the integrity of the gut lining is compromised, a condition known as **intestinal permeability** or **leaky gut** develops. The lining of the intestines consists of **intestinal epithelial cells** connected by **tight junctions**, which control what enters and leaves the bloodstream. When these tight junctions loosen, harmful substances—such as undigested food particles, toxins, and **pathogenic microorganisms**—can leak into the bloodstream, triggering an **immune response**.

This immune response involves the production of **inflammatory cytokines** and **antibodies**, leading to a cascade of immune system dysfunction. Over time, this **chronic inflammation** can result in the development of autoimmune conditions, where the immune system mistakenly attacks the body's own tissues.

Autoimmune Diseases and the Gut

Autoimmune diseases occur when the body's immune system starts attacking its own tissues, mistaking them for foreign invaders. In women, autoimmune diseases are disproportionately more common, and gut health plays a crucial role in their development. Research suggests that imbalances in the gut microbiome and increased intestinal permeability can lead to **autoimmunity**.

Why Autoimmune Diseases Are More Common in Women

Autoimmune diseases are significantly more prevalent in women than in men, with some conditions affecting women at a ratio of **9:1**. The reasons for this disparity are multifactorial and not fully understood, but several factors contribute:

1. **Hormonal Influences**: Hormones such as **estrogen** and **progesterone** can modulate immune function. These hormones are believed to enhance immune responses, which can contribute to the development of autoimmune diseases. For example, estrogen has been shown to increase the production of certain immune cells, which may explain why autoimmune conditions like **rheumatoid arthritis**, **lupus**, and **multiple sclerosis** are more common in women, particularly during their reproductive years.

2. **Genetics**: Women may be genetically predisposed to autoimmune diseases due to the presence of certain genes on the **X chromosome**, of which women have two, compared to men who only have one. This genetic factor may increase the likelihood of immune system dysregulation.

3. **Immune System Differences**: Women tend to have a more **active immune system** than men, which is why they are better equipped to fight off infections. However, this heightened immune response may also increase the risk of the immune system mistakenly attacking healthy cells, leading to autoimmune diseases.

Gut Health and Specific Autoimmune Diseases Common in Women

Several autoimmune diseases have been linked to **gut health dysfunction**, and many of these conditions are more common in women. Some of the most prevalent include:

1. Rheumatoid Arthritis (RA)

Rheumatoid arthritis is a chronic autoimmune condition that causes inflammation in the joints. Women are more likely to develop RA, especially between the ages of 30 and 60. **Leaky gut** has been implicated in RA, as gut permeability allows inflammatory substances to enter the bloodstream, which can trigger systemic inflammation and joint damage. The presence of certain gut bacteria may also influence the development and progression of RA, indicating the importance of maintaining a balanced microbiome.

2. Hashimoto's Thyroiditis

Hashimoto's thyroiditis is an autoimmune disease in which the immune system attacks the thyroid gland, leading to **hypothyroidism** (an underactive thyroid). Women are significantly more likely to develop Hashimoto's, and recent research has shown that **intestinal permeability** plays a key role in the onset of thyroid autoimmunity. A disrupted gut microbiome can lead to inflammation, which may contribute to thyroid dysfunction and the development of Hashimoto's disease.

3. Systemic Lupus Erythematosus (SLE)

Systemic lupus erythematosus (SLE), or lupus, is another autoimmune disease that disproportionately affects women, especially those of childbearing age. Lupus occurs when the immune system attacks various organs, including the skin, kidneys, and joints. Evidence suggests that **gut dysbiosis** plays a critical role in the development of lupus, as changes in the gut microbiome can lead to immune activation, which subsequently triggers autoimmunity.

4. Multiple Sclerosis (MS)

Multiple sclerosis is a disease in which the immune system attacks the **central nervous system**, leading to symptoms like weakness, numbness, and problems with coordination. Women are more likely to develop MS, and there is growing evidence linking **gut health** to MS. Studies suggest that **intestinal inflammation** and changes in the gut microbiome may contribute to the immune system's attack on the nervous system, thus increasing the risk of developing MS.

5. Celiac Disease

Celiac disease is an autoimmune disorder where the ingestion of **gluten** triggers an immune response that damages the small intestine. Women are more likely to develop celiac disease, and leaky gut is a key factor in its development. In those with celiac disease, gluten triggers the production of inflammatory cytokines, which increase intestinal permeability and damage the gut lining.

The Role of Diet in Modulating Gut Health and Immune Function

A **gut-friendly diet** is one of the most powerful tools for improving gut health and reducing inflammation. To promote a healthy gut microbiome and support immune system function, the following dietary practices are beneficial:

- **Anti-inflammatory foods**: Including omega-3 fatty acids (from fish, flaxseeds, and walnuts), colorful fruits and vegetables, and foods rich in polyphenols (like berries, green tea, and dark chocolate).
- **Probiotic-rich foods**: Fermented foods like **kimchi**, **sauerkraut**, **kefir**, and **yogurt** can help promote the growth of beneficial bacteria.
- **Prebiotic foods**: These include fiber-rich foods such as **garlic**, **onions**, **bananas**, and **asparagus**, which feed the good bacteria in the gut.
- **Avoiding gluten and processed foods**: For individuals with gut health issues, eliminating gluten and reducing processed foods can help improve gut permeability.

The Role of Gut Microbiota: The Importance of Gut Bacteria and Its Impact on Digestive and Mental Health

The human gut is home to an astonishingly diverse ecosystem of bacteria, viruses, fungi, and other microorganisms collectively known as the **gut microbiota**. These trillions of microorganisms play a vital role in maintaining **digestive health**, influencing **immune function**, and even impacting **mental health**. The balance or imbalance of this microbiota can be the difference between optimal health and the development of various health issues, including digestive disorders, chronic inflammation, and mood imbalances.

In this section, we will explore the crucial role of gut microbiota, how it influences both **digestive health** and **mental well-being**, and the ways in which an imbalance in these microbes—referred to as **dysbiosis**—can lead to significant health issues. Understanding the gut microbiota and its impact on overall health is particularly important for women, who are more susceptible to certain gut-related conditions and mental health challenges.

What is Gut Microbiota?

The **gut microbiota** is the vast collection of microorganisms living in your intestines, particularly in the colon. It consists of bacteria (which outnumber human cells), as well as viruses, fungi, and other microbes. These microbes are involved in various critical functions, including **digesting food, synthesizing essential vitamins,** and **training the immune system.**

The Role of Gut Microbiota in Digestive Health

A balanced and diverse gut microbiota is essential for efficient digestion and the absorption of nutrients. The microorganisms in your gut help break down complex food components that the body cannot digest on its own, such as **fiber, prebiotics,** and **complex carbohydrates**. These processes not only facilitate nutrient absorption but also produce **short-chain fatty acids (SCFAs)**, such as **butyrate**, which provide fuel for the cells of the colon and promote a healthy gut lining.

1. Digestion and Nutrient Absorption

Certain gut bacteria help break down **fibers** and **carbohydrates** that the human body cannot process directly. By fermenting these foods, gut bacteria produce gases and SCFAs, which nourish the gut lining and contribute to maintaining gut integrity. These SCFAs are also involved in the absorption of essential minerals such as **calcium, magnesium,** and **iron**. The microbiota thus plays a crucial role in ensuring your body gets the full nutritional benefit from food.

2. Maintaining Gut Integrity

The cells of the intestines are bound together by tight junctions that act as a protective barrier. This **intestinal barrier** prevents harmful substances, such as pathogens and toxins, from entering the bloodstream. **Healthy gut bacteria** produce metabolites that help reinforce these tight junctions, ensuring the integrity of the gut lining. When the microbiota is disrupted, these tight junctions can weaken, leading to **intestinal permeability** or **leaky gut**, where toxins and undigested food particles leak into the bloodstream, contributing to chronic inflammation and various digestive and autoimmune conditions.

3. Preventing Pathogen Overgrowth

A healthy balance of gut bacteria helps prevent the overgrowth of harmful bacteria and pathogens. The good bacteria occupy the space in the gut and compete with harmful microbes for nutrients and attachment sites. This competitive environment prevents the growth of potentially harmful organisms, such as **Clostridia, Salmonella,** and **Escherichia coli**. A disruption in the balance of good and bad bacteria—**dysbiosis**—can lead to the proliferation of harmful pathogens, resulting in conditions like **irritable bowel syndrome (IBS), Crohn's disease,** and **ulcerative colitis**.

The Impact of Gut Microbiota on Mental Health: The Gut-Brain Axis

In recent years, research has revealed a fascinating connection between the gut and the brain, often referred to as the **gut-brain axis**. This bi-directional communication network links the central nervous system (CNS) to the enteric nervous system (ENS), which governs the digestive system. The gut microbiota plays a pivotal role in modulating this connection, influencing mood, cognition, and mental health.

1. The Role of Gut Microbes in Neurotransmitter Production

Many of the same neurotransmitters that regulate mood and cognition—such as **serotonin, dopamine,** and **gamma-aminobutyric acid (GABA)**—are influenced by gut bacteria. It's estimated that around **90% of serotonin**, a neurotransmitter that stabilizes mood and contributes to feelings of well-being, is produced in the **gut**. Gut bacteria help synthesize and regulate serotonin production, influencing emotional states, stress responses, and even behavior.

- **Serotonin**: As mentioned, most of the body's serotonin is produced in the gut, and certain gut microbes can affect serotonin levels. Imbalances in serotonin are linked to mood disorders such as **depression** and **anxiety**.
- **Dopamine**: Similarly, dopamine, another mood-regulating neurotransmitter, is influenced by gut bacteria. Dopamine is involved in pleasure, motivation, and reward, and gut microbes may influence the reward systems in the brain.
- **GABA**: GABA is a key neurotransmitter that regulates **calmness** and **relaxation**. Some gut bacteria produce GABA, and imbalances in these bacteria may contribute to symptoms of **anxiety** and **stress**.

2. Gut Inflammation and Mental Health Disorders

Chronic gut inflammation, often caused by an imbalance in the gut microbiota, can affect the brain via the **gut-brain axis**, contributing to mood disturbances, **brain fog**, and other cognitive issues. Inflammatory molecules produced by harmful gut bacteria can travel to the brain and trigger inflammation there, leading to disruptions in normal brain function. This phenomenon is thought to contribute to various mental health conditions, such as:

- **Depression**: Dysbiosis has been associated with depression, as imbalances in the gut microbiota can lead to higher levels of **pro-inflammatory cytokines**, which may affect brain function and mood.
- **Anxiety**: A disrupted gut microbiota may increase the levels of **stress hormones** like **cortisol**, leading to heightened feelings of anxiety.
- **Cognitive Decline**: There is growing evidence that an imbalance in gut bacteria may contribute to neurodegenerative diseases such as **Alzheimer's disease** and **Parkinson's disease**. Inflammation and the buildup of **amyloid plaques** in the brain are thought to be linked to changes in the gut microbiome.

3. The Role of Gut Health in Stress and Anxiety

One of the most profound ways that gut health affects mental well-being is through its regulation of stress responses. When the gut microbiota is disrupted, it can lead to **increased stress hormone levels** (like **cortisol**) and **sympathetic nervous system activation**, which are associated with **anxiety** and **depression**. Additionally, gut dysbiosis can reduce the production of beneficial neurotransmitters like **GABA** and **serotonin**, which are essential for regulating calmness and mood.

Factors Affecting Gut Microbiota: Diet, Lifestyle, and Environment

A variety of factors influence the composition and diversity of your gut microbiota. Maintaining a **healthy gut** depends not only on what you eat but also on lifestyle choices and environmental factors that can either promote or disrupt a balanced microbiome.

1. Diet: The Gut's Most Powerful Influence

What you eat plays a major role in determining the health of your gut microbiota. A **fiber-rich diet** promotes the growth of beneficial bacteria, while a diet high in **sugar, processed foods**, and **artificial additives** can fuel harmful microbes and lead to dysbiosis. Foods like **fermented vegetables, yogurt, kefir**, and **kimchi** provide **probiotics** (live beneficial bacteria), while foods high in **fiber** (like whole grains, fruits, and vegetables) serve as **prebiotics**, feeding the good bacteria and helping them flourish.

2. Antibiotics and Medications

While antibiotics are essential for treating infections, their overuse can severely disrupt the gut microbiota by killing off both harmful and beneficial bacteria. This disruption can lead to dysbiosis and an increased risk of infections, digestive issues, and mental health problems.

3. Stress and Sleep

Chronic **stress** and poor **sleep hygiene** have both been shown to negatively impact the gut microbiota. Stress can increase gut permeability, allowing harmful substances to leak into the bloodstream and trigger inflammation. Similarly, insufficient sleep disrupts the production of **gut hormones** and impairs gut function, further contributing to gut dysbiosis.

4. Environmental Toxins

Environmental pollutants and toxins can also negatively affect gut health. Exposure to chemicals such as pesticides, heavy metals, and other environmental toxins may contribute to dysbiosis, leading to systemic inflammation, digestive issues, and mood disorders.

Inflammation and Leaky Gut: How Inflammation Caused by Leaky Gut Leads to Chronic Health Conditions, Including Chronic Fatigue, Skin Problems, and Autoimmune Disorders

Inflammation is the body's natural response to injury or infection. However, when it becomes chronic or uncontrolled, it can contribute to a wide range of health issues. One of the key drivers of chronic inflammation is **leaky gut syndrome**, a condition where the lining of the small intestine becomes damaged, allowing harmful substances like toxins, undigested food particles, and pathogens to leak into the bloodstream. This breakdown of the intestinal barrier triggers a cascade of immune responses, leading to widespread inflammation throughout the body. The resulting systemic inflammation can contribute to a variety of chronic health conditions, including **chronic fatigue**, **skin problems**, and **autoimmune disorders**—conditions that are often more prevalent and severe in women.

In this chapter, we'll delve into the process of how **leaky gut** leads to chronic inflammation and its connection to some of the most common and debilitating health issues. We'll explore how an imbalanced immune response and persistent inflammation can wreak havoc on the body, affecting everything from energy levels to the skin's appearance to the proper functioning of the immune system.

What is Inflammation and How Does it Relate to Leaky Gut?

Inflammation is part of the body's immune defense mechanism. When harmful substances enter the body, or when tissue damage occurs, the immune system responds by sending white blood cells and molecules like **cytokines** to the affected area. Acute inflammation is beneficial, as it helps the body heal. However, when inflammation becomes chronic—due to factors like persistent infections, toxin exposure, or gut imbalances—it can become a destructive force that damages tissues and organs, contributing to numerous health problems.

In a healthy gut, the lining of the intestines is made up of tightly bound cells that form a barrier to protect the bloodstream from harmful substances. However, in individuals with **leaky gut**, the intestinal lining becomes damaged, and the tight junctions between the gut cells loosen. This allows **toxins, undigested food particles**, and **pathogens** to pass through the gut lining and enter the bloodstream. The body perceives these foreign particles as threats, triggering an immune response. Over time, this constant low-level immune activation leads to chronic **systemic inflammation** that can spread throughout the body.

Chronic Fatigue and Leaky Gut: The Link Between Inflammation and Energy Levels

Chronic fatigue is one of the most common complaints among individuals with leaky gut, especially in women. The underlying cause of this fatigue is often tied to **inflammation** and the body's immune system constantly being in an activated state. When **toxins** and **bacterial particles** from the gut leak into the bloodstream, the immune system identifies them as invaders, triggering a persistent inflammatory response. This constant immune activation can cause the body to be in a prolonged state of stress, leading to the **overproduction of cortisol**, the stress hormone.

How Inflammation Contributes to Fatigue:

- **Increased Immune Activation**: As the immune system works to fight off the substances leaking from the gut, it releases inflammatory markers like **cytokines** (e.g., **TNF-alpha, IL-6**) that can directly interfere with the body's ability to function properly. These cytokines affect the brain, particularly the **hypothalamus**, the area responsible for regulating sleep-wake cycles, appetite, and energy balance. This disruption can lead to chronic fatigue and sleep disturbances.
- **Disrupted Sleep Patterns**: Inflammation also interferes with sleep quality, which further exacerbates fatigue. Research shows that pro-inflammatory cytokines disrupt **melatonin production** and **circadian rhythms**, making it harder to fall asleep and achieve restful, restorative sleep.
- **Mitochondrial Dysfunction**: Chronic inflammation can also affect the **mitochondria**, the energy-producing organelles in the

cells. This mitochondrial dysfunction reduces the body's ability to produce energy efficiently, leading to feelings of tiredness, low energy, and weakness.

Skin Problems and Leaky Gut: How Inflammation Leads to Chronic Skin Conditions

Another area where leaky gut and chronic inflammation have a profound impact is on **skin health**. The skin is often considered a reflection of internal health, and when systemic inflammation is present, it manifests on the skin in a variety of forms. Conditions like **eczema, rosacea, acne, psoriasis**, and other inflammatory skin disorders are common among individuals with leaky gut.

How Inflammation Affects Skin Health:

- **Skin Irritation and Sensitivity**: Chronic systemic inflammation can increase the body's production of inflammatory molecules that affect the skin, leading to heightened sensitivity and irritation. The immune system's response to leaky gut can trigger flare-ups of skin conditions like eczema and psoriasis. These conditions cause red, inflamed, itchy, and sometimes cracked skin, significantly impacting a person's quality of life.
- **Acne and Rosacea**: Inflammatory cytokines can also stimulate **sebaceous gland** activity, leading to excess oil production and clogged pores, which can worsen **acne**. Additionally, the inflammation caused by leaky gut can trigger or worsen **rosacea**, a condition characterized by redness, swelling, and visible blood vessels, typically around the face.
- **Accelerated Aging**: Chronic inflammation is a key factor in **premature aging**. When the body experiences prolonged systemic inflammation, it can lead to the breakdown of **collagen** and **elastin** fibers in the skin. This damage results in **wrinkles, fine lines**, and loss of skin elasticity, making the skin look older and more worn down.

Autoimmune Disorders and Leaky Gut: How Inflammation Disrupts Immune Function

One of the most concerning consequences of leaky gut and chronic inflammation is the potential for developing **autoimmune disorders**. In a healthy immune system, the body is able to distinguish between its own healthy tissues and foreign invaders. However, in individuals with leaky gut, the constant entry of toxins and undigested food particles into the bloodstream can confuse the immune system, triggering it to attack the body's own cells. This process is known as **autoimmunity**, and it leads to a variety of chronic conditions.

How Leaky Gut Contributes to Autoimmune Diseases:

- **Molecular Mimicry**: In some cases, the immune system mistakes the body's own tissues for foreign invaders due to **molecular mimicry**. When the immune system encounters a substance that closely resembles the body's cells—often due to undigested food particles or **gut bacteria**—it may begin attacking those tissues. This process can lead to diseases like **rheumatoid arthritis, multiple sclerosis, type 1 diabetes**, and **Hashimoto's thyroiditis**.

- **Chronic Immune Activation**: Persistent inflammation due to leaky gut keeps the immune system constantly activated, leading to the development of autoimmune conditions. Over time, this activation exhausts the immune system, making it more susceptible to attacking healthy cells, tissues, and organs.

- **Specific Autoimmune Conditions in Women**: Autoimmune diseases are more common in women, and conditions like **lupus, rheumatoid arthritis**, and **Graves' disease** are often exacerbated by the underlying inflammation associated with leaky gut. In some cases, the autoimmune response may also involve hormone-related triggers, further complicating the condition.

Managing Chronic Inflammation and Leaky Gut: Solutions and Lifestyle Adjustments

While leaky gut and its resulting inflammation can lead to a range of chronic health conditions, there are steps you can take to manage inflammation and promote gut healing. Addressing the root cause of leaky gut—intestinal permeability—is key to improving overall health and reducing the risk of chronic conditions.

1. Anti-inflammatory Diet: An anti-inflammatory diet rich in omega-3 fatty acids, antioxidants, fiber, and lean proteins can help reduce

inflammation in the body. Avoiding processed foods, refined sugars, and gluten can prevent exacerbating inflammation and encourage gut healing.

2. Gut-Healing Nutrients: Nutrients like L-glutamine, collagen, zinc, and probiotics help restore the integrity of the gut lining, reduce inflammation, and support the healing of leaky gut. Eating bone broth, fermented foods, and high-fiber vegetables can help nourish the gut and balance the microbiome.

3. Stress Reduction and Sleep: Managing stress through practices like yoga, meditation, or deep breathing can help regulate cortisol levels and reduce inflammation. Additionally, prioritizing restorative sleep ensures the body has the time it needs to heal and repair.

4. Supplements: Certain supplements, such as curcumin (from turmeric), omega-3s, and vitamin D, are known for their anti-inflammatory properties and can help reduce chronic inflammation associated with leaky gut.

Chapter 3: The Key Causes of Leaky Gut in Women: Hormones, Diet, and Lifestyle

Leaky gut syndrome is a multifaceted condition, and for many women, the causes are often intertwined with hormonal fluctuations, dietary habits, and lifestyle factors. Understanding these triggers is key to addressing leaky gut, as it allows for targeted interventions that can heal the gut and restore balance to the body. In this chapter, we will explore the primary factors contributing to the development of leaky gut in women, highlighting how **hormonal imbalances, poor diet**, and **stressful lifestyles** can each play a role in disrupting gut health.

1. Hormonal Imbalances and Leaky Gut in Women

Hormones are powerful regulators of bodily functions, and their fluctuations throughout a woman's life—during menstruation, pregnancy, and menopause—can significantly impact gut health. Hormonal imbalances, particularly those related to **estrogen**, **progesterone**, and **cortisol**, can compromise the integrity of the gut lining, leading to **intestinal permeability** (leaky gut).

Estrogen and Leaky Gut

Estrogen is a key hormone in regulating female reproductive health, but its levels also have a significant impact on the gut. **High levels of estrogen**, particularly during pregnancy or in women using hormone replacement therapy (HRT), can promote **intestinal permeability** by disrupting the balance of the gut microbiome. Research suggests that estrogen may alter the tight junctions between intestinal cells, weakening the gut lining and making it more vulnerable to leakage.

- **Pregnancy**: During pregnancy, estrogen and progesterone levels rise significantly, which can affect gut motility and microbiota composition. These changes may predispose women to digestive issues like bloating, constipation, and gas—symptoms often linked to leaky gut.
- **Hormonal Contraceptives**: Birth control pills and other hormonal contraceptives that alter estrogen and progesterone levels may also contribute to leaky gut. These medications have been shown to affect gut permeability and may increase inflammation in some women.

Progesterone and Leaky Gut

Progesterone is another hormone that plays a crucial role in gut health. It has a calming effect on the digestive tract, helping to regulate gut motility and inflammation. However, **low progesterone levels**—which are common during perimenopause and menopause—can contribute to **gut dysbiosis** (an imbalance in gut bacteria), leading to a more permeable gut lining. This, in turn, can promote inflammation and worsen symptoms of leaky gut.

- **Perimenopause and Menopause**: As estrogen and progesterone levels fluctuate during perimenopause and menopause, women often experience a decline in gut health. Reduced progesterone can result in increased gut inflammation, bloating, and digestive discomfort, all of which can contribute to leaky gut.

Cortisol and Stress

Cortisol, the body's primary stress hormone, plays a significant role in gut health. Chronic stress leads to **elevated cortisol levels**, which can disrupt the gut lining and increase intestinal permeability. When cortisol is chronically high, it can impair the ability of the gut to heal and maintain

its barrier function, making the gut more susceptible to leaky gut.
- **Stress Response**: In stressful situations, cortisol directs the body's resources toward dealing with immediate danger, including suppressing non-essential functions like digestion. Over time, this chronic stress can lead to imbalanced gut bacteria, inflammation, and impaired intestinal health.
- **Cortisol Imbalances**: Women are particularly susceptible to the effects of chronic stress, with higher rates of anxiety and depression that can lead to cortisol dysregulation. This creates a vicious cycle where stress exacerbates gut permeability, which, in turn, worsens stress-related symptoms.

2. Diet and Leaky Gut in Women

Diet is one of the most significant contributors to the development of leaky gut. Certain foods can directly impact the health of the gut lining, promote inflammation, and imbalance the gut microbiome. Women, in particular, may be more vulnerable to dietary factors due to their hormonal fluctuations, nutritional needs, and lifestyle choices.

Processed Foods and Sugar

Diets high in **processed foods**, **refined sugars**, and **trans fats** are major contributors to leaky gut. These foods promote inflammation in the gut, disrupt the balance of the gut microbiota, and weaken the gut lining. Sugar, for example, feeds **bad bacteria** in the gut, allowing them to proliferate and overpower **beneficial bacteria**.
- **Sugar and Inflammation**: A high-sugar diet promotes the release of **pro-inflammatory cytokines**, which contribute to intestinal permeability. Women who consume high levels of sugary snacks, sodas, and processed foods are particularly vulnerable to gut inflammation and leaky gut.
- **Gluten Sensitivity**: Women may also be more likely to develop **gluten intolerance**, which can contribute to leaky gut. Gluten has been shown to increase intestinal permeability in sensitive individuals, especially those with **celiac disease** or **non-celiac gluten sensitivity**. Even without full-blown gluten intolerance, regular consumption of gluten can damage the gut lining in some women, triggering inflammation and gut leakage.

Low Fiber Intake

Fiber is essential for a healthy gut. A diet low in **fiber-rich fruits, vegetables,** and **whole grains** can contribute to an imbalance in the gut microbiota, making it more difficult to maintain a healthy gut lining. Fiber is a prebiotic that feeds **good bacteria**, and a lack of it can lead to overgrowth of harmful microbes that disrupt gut health.

- **Gut Flora Imbalance**: Low fiber intake has been linked to dysbiosis, which is a shift in the composition of the gut microbiota that promotes the growth of harmful bacteria and reduces beneficial bacteria. This imbalance can lead to inflammation, gut permeability, and the development of leaky gut.

Food Sensitivities and Leaky Gut

Women are more likely to experience food sensitivities or intolerances, particularly to dairy, gluten, and processed foods. These sensitivities can irritate the gut lining and trigger an inflammatory response. For example, **lactose intolerance** can lead to gut irritation and inflammation, exacerbating leaky gut symptoms.

- **Dairy and Gut Health**: Dairy products, especially those high in fat, can be difficult to digest for some individuals. In women with lactose intolerance or sensitivity to casein (the protein found in dairy), consuming dairy can lead to bloating, gas, and intestinal inflammation, all of which contribute to leaky gut.

3. Lifestyle Factors Contributing to Leaky Gut

In addition to hormonal fluctuations and diet, various lifestyle factors can also play a significant role in the development and progression of leaky gut in women. These include chronic stress, lack of sleep, lack of physical activity, and environmental toxins.

Chronic Stress

As mentioned earlier, chronic stress is a major contributor to leaky gut. Women are particularly susceptible to stress-related gut issues due to their multi-tasking roles, caregiving responsibilities, and work-life balance challenges. Prolonged stress leads to sustained **high cortisol levels**, which disrupt the gut barrier, leading to increased intestinal permeability.

- **Emotional Stress**: In addition to physical stress, **emotional stress** can also take a toll on gut health. Women, who are more likely to experience emotional stress related to relationships, work, and family, may experience more profound impacts on their gut microbiome and intestinal integrity.

Lack of Sleep

Sleep deprivation has a direct impact on the health of the gut. Chronic lack of sleep has been shown to alter the gut microbiome and increase gut permeability. When women do not get enough **quality sleep**, the body's ability to repair and regenerate the gut lining is impaired, leading to increased inflammation and intestinal dysfunction.

- **Sleep and Immune Function**: Sleep is essential for regulating the immune system and maintaining gut health. Women who experience **insomnia, shift work**, or **poor sleep quality** are at higher risk of developing gut-related issues, including leaky gut.

Environmental Toxins

Environmental toxins, such as **pesticides, pollutants,** and **chemicals** in personal care products, can contribute to leaky gut by triggering inflammation in the body. These toxins often interfere with the gut's ability to maintain its protective barrier, leading to increased permeability and gut dysbiosis.

- **Endocrine Disruptors**: Women are more likely to be exposed to **endocrine-disrupting chemicals** (EDCs), which can interfere with hormonal balance and contribute to leaky gut. These chemicals are found in many household products, including cleaning supplies, plastics, and cosmetics.

Estrogen Dominance: The Role of Estrogen Dominance in Women's Gut Health and How It Exacerbates Leaky Gut

Estrogen dominance is a condition that occurs when there is an imbalance between estrogen and progesterone in the body, often resulting in higher-than-normal levels of estrogen relative to progesterone. This hormonal imbalance is common in women, especially as they approach perimenopause, menopause, or due to external factors such as birth control or hormone replacement therapy (HRT). Estrogen dominance can have a significant impact on various aspects of health, and one area where it plays a critical role is **gut health**. In particular, it can worsen the symptoms of **leaky gut syndrome** by exacerbating gut inflammation, disrupting the gut microbiome, and impairing the gut's ability to heal.

In this section, we will dive deep into how **estrogen dominance** affects the gut and why it is such a crucial factor in the development of leaky gut in women. We will explore the connection between estrogen dominance and the gut lining, the inflammatory response, and how this hormonal imbalance may contribute to intestinal permeability.

1. What is Estrogen Dominance?

Estrogen dominance refers to a state in which the body has higher levels of **estrogen** relative to **progesterone**, even though the total amount of estrogen may be normal or elevated. This imbalance often occurs in the following situations:

- **Perimenopause and Menopause**: As women approach menopause, their estrogen levels fluctuate and may be higher compared to progesterone, especially in the early stages of perimenopause. This can lead to symptoms of estrogen dominance.
- **Hormonal Contraceptives and Hormone Replacement Therapy (HRT)**: Birth control pills and HRT, which are designed to increase estrogen levels, can sometimes cause an estrogen-progesterone imbalance, contributing to estrogen dominance.
- **Environmental Estrogen Exposure (Xenoestrogens)**: Women may also experience estrogen dominance due to **xenoestrogens**, which are synthetic compounds found in plastics, pesticides, and personal care products that mimic estrogen in the body. Prolonged exposure to these chemicals can elevate estrogen levels and disrupt the natural hormone balance.

When estrogen dominance occurs, the body is left with too much estrogen circulating relative to progesterone. Progesterone is a hormone that counteracts some of the effects of estrogen, and without enough progesterone to balance estrogen's influence, the body can experience a cascade of symptoms and health issues, including its impact on gut health.

2. Estrogen and the Gut: How Estrogen Affects Intestinal Permeability

Estrogen has a profound influence on gut function and integrity, but when in excess, it can significantly impair the health of the gastrointestinal system. The relationship between estrogen and the gut is complex and bidirectional. On the one hand, **estrogen** helps maintain gut motility and supports the growth of beneficial gut bacteria. On the other hand, excess estrogen—especially in the form of estrogen dominance—can lead to a breakdown of the intestinal barrier, exacerbating **leaky gut syndrome**.

Estrogen's Impact on Gut Lining and Permeability

The gut lining is made up of tightly connected cells that form a **protective barrier**, preventing harmful substances, toxins, and pathogens from entering the bloodstream. These connections are maintained by tight junctions, which are small protein complexes that hold the cells together. **Excess estrogen** can influence the tight junctions in the gut lining, making them more vulnerable to disruption. When these junctions become compromised, it results in increased **intestinal permeability**, or **leaky gut**.

- **Estrogen Receptors in the Gut**: Estrogen has receptors in the cells lining the gut, which means that estrogen can directly affect gut health. When estrogen levels are high, it can increase the permeability of the gut lining by altering the structure and function of these receptors, leading to a weakened gut barrier.
- **Leaky Gut and Estrogen Dominance**: Research has shown that high levels of estrogen can trigger the breakdown of tight junctions in the gut, leading to **increased gut permeability**. This allows toxins, undigested food particles, and harmful bacteria to pass into the bloodstream, which can then trigger systemic inflammation and immune responses that exacerbate symptoms of leaky gut.

The Gut-Immune System Connection

A compromised gut lining due to estrogen dominance can also have far-reaching effects on the **immune system**. The gut is home to approximately 70-80% of the body's immune cells, which are responsible for defending against harmful invaders and regulating inflammation. When estrogen causes the gut lining to become permeable, it can allow the immune system to become overactive, leading to **systemic inflammation** and the development of autoimmune conditions. This is especially concerning for women who are already predisposed to autoimmune diseases such as **Hashimoto's thyroiditis, rheumatoid arthritis,** or **lupus**.

3. Estrogen Dominance and Gut Inflammation

One of the most significant consequences of estrogen dominance is the promotion of **gut inflammation**. Chronic low-grade inflammation is often present in women with estrogen dominance and is a key factor in the development of leaky gut. High estrogen levels can induce inflammatory cytokines and disrupt the balance of the gut microbiota, further contributing to an inflamed, permeable gut.

Chronic Inflammation and Leaky Gut

When estrogen dominance causes an increase in gut inflammation, the gut becomes more susceptible to damage, leading to **intestinal permeability**. This inflammation not only damages the gut lining but also triggers the release of **pro-inflammatory cytokines** that can affect other organs and systems in the body. This cascade of inflammation can contribute to the development of chronic health conditions, including:

- **Chronic fatigue**
- **Bloating**
- **Skin conditions (e.g., acne, eczema)**
- **Autoimmune disorders**
- **Digestive discomfort**

Gut Microbiome Imbalance

Estrogen dominance can also affect the balance of the **gut microbiota**—the community of bacteria, viruses, fungi, and other microorganisms that live in the gut. A healthy microbiome is crucial for maintaining gut integrity and preventing leaky gut. However, **imbalanced estrogen levels** can promote the growth of harmful bacteria and yeast in the gut while suppressing the beneficial microbes that help maintain a healthy barrier.

- **Dysbiosis**: The imbalance in the gut microbiota, known as **dysbiosis**, is a hallmark of estrogen dominance. When estrogen levels are too high, it can create an environment that favors harmful bacteria and yeast, further exacerbating gut permeability and inflammation.

4. Symptoms of Estrogen Dominance and Their Impact on Gut Health

The symptoms of estrogen dominance in women are wide-ranging and can manifest both in the gut and throughout the body. Some of the most common signs of estrogen dominance that contribute to leaky gut include:

Digestive Symptoms

- **Bloating**: Estrogen dominance often leads to water retention and bloating, which can be exacerbated by the **inflammation** caused by leaky gut.
- **Constipation or Diarrhea**: High estrogen levels can affect gut motility, leading to **irregular bowel movements**, which may worsen if gut permeability is increased.
- **Gas and Indigestion**: Estrogen dominance may contribute to discomfort, including **gas** and **indigestion**, due to its impact on gut function and microbial balance.

Hormonal Imbalances

- **Irregular Periods**: Estrogen dominance can disrupt the menstrual cycle, leading to **heavy periods, spotting**, or **PMS**. These symptoms are closely tied to estrogen's influence on the gut, as hormonal imbalances in the reproductive system often coincide with gut disturbances.
- **Mood Swings and Fatigue**: The hormonal fluctuations associated with estrogen dominance can cause **mood swings**, **anxiety**, and **fatigue**, all of which are often linked to the inflammatory effects of leaky gut on the nervous system.

5. Addressing Estrogen Dominance and Supporting Gut Health

To address estrogen dominance and support gut health, women need to take a multi-faceted approach that includes dietary changes, stress management, and hormonal balancing.

- **Reducing Estrogenic Exposure**: Minimizing exposure to environmental toxins (xenoestrogens) and managing external hormone treatments (such as birth control and HRT) can help regulate estrogen levels.
- **Supporting Hormonal Balance**: Incorporating **phytoestrogens** (natural plant-based estrogens) and **progesterone support** (e.g., through supplements or diet) can help balance estrogen levels and reduce estrogen dominance.
- **Gut-Healing Diet**: A gut-healing diet rich in **fiber, fermented foods**, and **anti-inflammatory nutrients** can help restore balance to the gut microbiome, reduce inflammation, and improve gut barrier function.
- **Stress Reduction**: Chronic stress management through mindfulness, meditation, exercise, and relaxation techniques can help regulate cortisol levels and support hormonal balance.

Food Sensitivities: Understanding Which Foods Trigger Leaky Gut and How Food Allergies and Intolerances Play a Role

Food sensitivities, allergies, and intolerances are common culprits in the development and exacerbation of **leaky gut syndrome**. When the gut becomes overly permeable, or "leaky," it allows undigested food particles, toxins, and microbes to enter the bloodstream, which can trigger an immune response and lead to inflammation throughout the body. For women in particular, certain foods can act as triggers for leaky gut, leading to digestive issues, autoimmune flare-ups, skin problems, and other systemic symptoms.

In this section, we will explore how **food sensitivities** contribute to the development of **leaky gut**, identify common foods that can worsen gut health, and explain the mechanisms behind food allergies and intolerances. Understanding this relationship can help you make informed dietary choices and support your gut healing process.

1. The Mechanisms of Food Sensitivities and Leaky Gut

The link between food sensitivities and **leaky gut** is complex, but it primarily revolves around the immune system, gut inflammation, and gut permeability.

How Food Sensitivities Impact Gut Health

When you consume a food that your body is sensitive to, the immune system recognizes it as harmful and triggers an inflammatory response. This immune activation can directly impact the gut lining, causing the **tight junctions** between the cells of the intestinal wall to loosen. These tight junctions normally act as a barrier, preventing larger particles from passing into the bloodstream. However, when food sensitivities or intolerances are present, this barrier function becomes impaired, leading to **intestinal permeability** or **leaky gut**.

- **Inflammatory Cytokines**: When the immune system reacts to an offending food, it releases **inflammatory cytokines** that increase gut permeability. These cytokines not only damage the gut lining but can also promote **systemic inflammation**, which affects organs and tissues throughout the body.
- **Immune System Activation**: The body's immune system often responds to food sensitivities by producing antibodies, such as **IgG (Immunoglobulin G)**, against certain food proteins. This immune reaction leads to chronic inflammation in the gut, contributing to the breakdown of the intestinal barrier and the onset of leaky gut.

Food Allergies and Leaky Gut

Food allergies are different from food sensitivities but can have a similarly destructive impact on gut health. In a food allergy, the immune system overreacts to a harmless food protein, triggering an immediate response, often including symptoms such as **hives, swelling, nausea, and difficulty breathing**. While food allergies are usually more severe and acute in nature, they also contribute to leaky gut by causing an inflammatory cascade that damages the intestinal lining.

- **IgE-Dependent Reactions**: Food allergies typically involve the production of **IgE antibodies**, which are responsible for triggering an immediate allergic reaction. This reaction leads to an influx of histamine and other inflammatory mediators, further compromising the integrity of the gut lining and promoting leaky gut.
- **Chronic Inflammation**: Repeated exposure to allergenic foods over time can lead to chronic inflammation in the gut. This

sustained inflammation weakens the gut barrier, resulting in leaky gut syndrome.

Food Intolerances and Their Role

Food intolerances, such as **lactose intolerance** or **gluten intolerance**, do not typically involve an immune response like food allergies. Instead, they occur when the body has difficulty digesting certain foods or food components. While the immune system isn't directly involved in food intolerances, the digestive disturbances they cause can still impair gut health and contribute to **intestinal permeability**.

- **Lactose Intolerance**: Individuals with lactose intolerance lack the enzyme **lactase**, which is necessary to break down lactose, the sugar found in dairy products. When lactose is not properly digested, it can ferment in the gut, leading to **gas, bloating, and diarrhea**. This fermentation process can contribute to gut inflammation, weaken the gut lining, and increase permeability.
- **Gluten Intolerance**: Gluten, a protein found in wheat, barley, and rye, is another common trigger for leaky gut. For those with gluten intolerance or **non-celiac gluten sensitivity**, gluten can lead to inflammation in the gut, disrupting the tight junctions between intestinal cells and promoting leaky gut.

2. Common Foods that Trigger Leaky Gut

Certain foods are known to exacerbate leaky gut by triggering inflammatory responses, damaging the gut lining, and promoting an imbalance in the gut microbiota. Here are some of the most common foods that can contribute to leaky gut, especially in women who may already be dealing with hormonal imbalances or autoimmune conditions.

1. Gluten

Gluten, found in wheat, barley, and rye, is a well-known irritant for individuals with **celiac disease** and **gluten intolerance**. Even for those who don't have a diagnosed gluten sensitivity, consuming gluten can still cause mild gut inflammation and permeability in some individuals, contributing to the development or worsening of leaky gut.

- **Gluten and Gut Inflammation**: Gluten has been shown to trigger an immune response that leads to gut inflammation, even in people who don't have celiac disease. In genetically predisposed individuals, gluten can bind to the **zonulin** protein, which regulates the tight junctions in the gut. This binding causes the junctions to loosen, allowing harmful particles to leak into the bloodstream.

2. Dairy

Dairy products, especially **milk** and **cheese**, can cause digestive discomfort in many individuals, particularly those with **lactose intolerance**. The inability to break down lactose leads to gas, bloating, and diarrhea, which can irritate the gut lining and exacerbate leaky gut symptoms.

- **Inflammation from Dairy**: For some women, dairy can also cause an inflammatory response in the body, even without the presence of lactose intolerance. This is due to the proteins found in dairy, such as **casein** and **whey**, which can act as allergens and trigger inflammation in the digestive tract.

3. Processed Foods and Sugars

Highly processed foods and refined sugars can cause an imbalance in the gut microbiome, promoting the growth of harmful bacteria and yeast, which in turn contribute to gut inflammation and leaky gut. Diets high in refined sugar can cause spikes in **insulin**, leading to **inflammation** throughout the body, including in the gut.

- **Sugar and Dysbiosis**: High sugar intake has been linked to **dysbiosis**, an imbalance in the gut microbiota, where harmful bacteria outnumber beneficial ones. Dysbiosis weakens the gut barrier, leading to increased intestinal permeability.

4. Artificial Sweeteners

Artificial sweeteners like **aspartame**, **sucralose**, and **saccharin** are often used in processed foods and beverages as sugar substitutes. While these sweeteners may be calorie-free, they can disrupt gut health by altering the microbiome and increasing intestinal permeability.

- **Artificial Sweeteners and Gut Microbiota**: Some studies suggest that artificial sweeteners can negatively affect the balance of gut bacteria, promoting the growth of pathogenic organisms that contribute to **gut inflammation** and leaky gut.

5. Nightshades

Nightshade vegetables, such as **tomatoes, potatoes, eggplant,** and **peppers**, contain **solanine**, a compound that can be irritating to some individuals, particularly those with **autoimmune conditions**. While nightshades are generally healthy foods, they can trigger an immune response that exacerbates leaky gut symptoms in sensitive individuals.

- **Solanine and Gut Health**: Solanine can cause inflammation in the digestive tract, leading to irritation and damage to the gut lining. For individuals with autoimmune conditions, nightshades can worsen symptoms by increasing gut permeability and promoting systemic inflammation.

6. Alcohol

Alcohol, particularly in excess, can be extremely damaging to gut health. It irritates the gut lining, promotes inflammation, and disrupts the gut microbiota, leading to **intestinal permeability** and exacerbating the symptoms of leaky gut.

- **Alcohol and Gut Permeability**: Alcohol consumption can increase the expression of **zonulin**, the protein that regulates tight junctions in the gut. This leads to a breakdown of the intestinal barrier, allowing toxins and other harmful substances to leak into the bloodstream.

3. How to Manage Food Sensitivities and Heal Leaky Gut

If you suspect that food sensitivities are contributing to your leaky gut, the first step is to identify and eliminate trigger foods from your diet. A food journal or **elimination diet** can be helpful in pinpointing the specific foods that exacerbate your symptoms.

- **Elimination Diet**: An elimination diet involves removing potential trigger foods (such as gluten, dairy, sugar, and processed foods) from your diet for a few weeks and then reintroducing them one at a time to see if symptoms worsen.
- **Gut-Healing Foods**: Focus on nutrient-dense, anti-inflammatory foods that support gut health, such as **bone broth, fermented foods** (e.g., kefir, sauerkraut, kimchi), **fiber-rich vegetables,** and **healthy fats** (e.g., avocado, olive oil).
- **Gut Healing Supplements**: Supplements such as **L-**

glutamine, collagen peptides, and **probiotics** can help repair the gut lining and restore a healthy microbiome.

Chronic Stress and Leaky Gut: How Cortisol Levels from Chronic Stress Can Worsen Gut Permeability

In today's fast-paced world, chronic stress has become an all-too-common part of life. Whether it's due to work pressures, family demands, financial worries, or health concerns, stress is an unavoidable aspect of modern living. However, what many don't realize is that stress not only affects our mental and emotional well-being but can also wreak havoc on our **physical health**, particularly our **gut health**.

One of the most important ways chronic stress impacts our body is through the **hormone cortisol**. Cortisol, often referred to as the "stress hormone," plays a crucial role in the body's fight-or-flight response and regulates several vital bodily functions. However, when cortisol levels remain elevated for prolonged periods due to chronic stress, it can lead to **gut dysfunction** and contribute significantly to **leaky gut syndrome**.

In this section, we will explore how **chronic stress** elevates cortisol levels, the mechanisms by which cortisol contributes to **intestinal permeability**, and the cascading effects of chronic stress on gut health. Understanding the relationship between stress and leaky gut is essential for women, as hormonal fluctuations and stress often go hand in hand, exacerbating gut issues and contributing to a host of chronic health problems.

1. Understanding Cortisol and Its Role in Stress

Cortisol is a steroid hormone produced by the adrenal glands in response to stress. When you face a stressful situation, whether physical or emotional, your **sympathetic nervous system** activates and signals the adrenal glands to release cortisol into your bloodstream. This is part of the **fight-or-flight response**, which prepares the body to deal with perceived threats by increasing alertness, boosting energy, and suppressing non-essential functions.

While cortisol plays a critical role in the body's immediate response to stress, prolonged activation due to chronic stress leads to **elevated cortisol levels** over time. This can have widespread effects on various bodily systems, including digestion and the immune system.

The Ideal vs. Chronic Stress Response
- **Acute Stress**: In short bursts, cortisol is beneficial. It helps you stay alert, focused, and energized in moments of danger or urgency. After the stressful event passes, cortisol levels should return to normal, allowing the body to relax and restore balance.
- **Chronic Stress**: When stress is ongoing, such as in chronic work pressure or personal struggles, the body remains in a heightened state of alert. Cortisol remains elevated, disrupting numerous bodily systems and potentially leading to **chronic inflammation** and a breakdown of various physiological functions, including those involved in **gut health.**

2. How Cortisol Contributes to Leaky Gut

When cortisol levels are chronically elevated, they can trigger a cascade of biological events that lead to **intestinal permeability** — more commonly known as **leaky gut**. Here's how chronic stress and elevated cortisol disrupt the gut:

1. Cortisol and Tight Junctions

The lining of your gut is made up of epithelial cells that are tightly bound together by **tight junctions**. These tight junctions form a barrier that prevents harmful substances such as bacteria, toxins, and undigested food particles from leaking into the bloodstream. However, when cortisol is chronically elevated, it can interfere with the integrity of these tight junctions, causing them to loosen and allow unwanted substances to slip through.

- **Disruption of Tight Junction Proteins**: Chronic cortisol secretion has been shown to reduce the expression of proteins involved in maintaining tight junction integrity, such as **occludin** and **zonulin**. The breakdown of these proteins leads to a weakened gut barrier, allowing harmful substances to penetrate the bloodstream and trigger **immune system activation.**

2. Chronic Inflammation

Chronic stress and the elevated cortisol levels that come with it can cause long-term inflammation in the body. **Inflammation** is a key player in the development of leaky gut. Cortisol, while initially anti-inflammatory in acute situations, becomes counterproductive when present for long periods.

- **Cytokine Release**: Cortisol helps to regulate inflammation by suppressing the production of **pro-inflammatory cytokines** in acute stress situations. However, when stress is chronic, cortisol's anti-inflammatory effect becomes less effective, and inflammation persists. This ongoing inflammation weakens the gut lining and contributes to the development of leaky gut.
- **Gut Inflammation**: Elevated cortisol can also stimulate the release of other inflammatory mediators like **histamine**, which further exacerbates gut inflammation, damaging the intestinal lining. This creates a vicious cycle, where inflammation leads to gut permeability, and leaky gut, in turn, promotes further inflammation in the body.

3. Gut Microbiome Imbalance

The gut microbiome, made up of trillions of beneficial bacteria, plays a critical role in maintaining a healthy gut barrier. However, chronic stress and high cortisol levels can disrupt the balance of the microbiome, favoring the growth of **pathogenic bacteria** and reducing the abundance of **beneficial bacteria**.

- **Dysbiosis and Leaky Gut**: Dysbiosis, or an imbalance in the gut microbiome, has been strongly linked to increased intestinal permeability. The overgrowth of harmful bacteria and the depletion of beneficial bacteria can lead to inflammation and further damage to the gut lining, exacerbating leaky gut symptoms.

4. Impaired Digestive Function

Chronic stress and elevated cortisol can impair several digestive functions, including **gastric acid secretion, enzyme production**, and **intestinal motility**. This can result in inadequate digestion, leading to the malabsorption of nutrients and an increased load of undigested food particles that can irritate the gut lining.

- **Reduced Gastric Acid**: Chronic stress can reduce the production of **stomach acid**, which is crucial for breaking down food and killing harmful pathogens. Low stomach acid can lead to **bacterial overgrowth** and an increased risk of **gut**

infections, further promoting leaky gut.
- **Slowed Gut Motility**: Cortisol can also slow down the motility of the intestines, leading to **constipation, bloating,** and **gas**. This sluggish digestion allows food to sit in the gut longer, which can promote the overgrowth of harmful bacteria, further damaging the gut lining and increasing permeability.

3. The Impact of Chronic Stress on Gut Health in Women

For women, the relationship between chronic stress and gut health is often compounded by **hormonal fluctuations** that are unique to the female body. Stress, combined with hormonal imbalances during menstruation, pregnancy, and menopause, can significantly worsen the effects of leaky gut.

- **Estrogen and Cortisol**: Estrogen, the primary female sex hormone, has a significant relationship with cortisol. **Estrogen dominance** or fluctuations in estrogen levels can affect the body's ability to manage stress and cortisol production. High cortisol levels can exacerbate **gut inflammation** in women who are already dealing with **estrogen imbalances**, leading to a double-whammy for gut health.
- **Menstrual Cycle and Stress**: The menstrual cycle also plays a role in how stress affects gut health. During certain phases, particularly the **luteal phase**, women may be more susceptible to stress and cortisol spikes. This can exacerbate leaky gut symptoms like **bloating, irregular bowel movements**, and **fatigue**.
- **Adrenal Fatigue**: Chronic stress can also lead to **adrenal fatigue**, a condition in which the adrenal glands become depleted and are no longer able to produce adequate cortisol. This can result in a state of **cortisol imbalance**, where the body's ability to manage stress is impaired, and inflammation and gut permeability increase.

4. Managing Stress to Support Gut Health

Managing chronic stress is one of the most effective ways to prevent or heal leaky gut. By lowering cortisol levels, you can reduce inflammation, improve gut permeability, and support overall gut health.

Stress-Reduction Techniques

Here are some strategies to help manage chronic stress and support gut healing:

- **Mindfulness Meditation**: Mindfulness and meditation can help reduce the body's stress response and lower cortisol levels. Even just a few minutes of deep breathing or meditation each day can have significant benefits.
- **Exercise**: Regular exercise is a natural way to reduce cortisol levels and improve overall well-being. Activities like walking, yoga, or swimming can be particularly beneficial for managing stress.
- **Adequate Sleep**: Quality sleep is essential for cortisol regulation. Prioritize restful sleep to help the body recover from stress and lower cortisol production.
- **Nutrition**: Eating a balanced diet rich in **anti-inflammatory foods**, including **omega-3 fatty acids** (from fish or flaxseed), **fiber** (from vegetables and fruits), and **probiotics** (from fermented foods), can help reduce inflammation and improve gut health.
- **Therapy and Support**: Cognitive Behavioral Therapy (CBT) or counseling can help address the root causes of chronic stress and provide coping mechanisms for dealing with life's challenges.

By reducing chronic stress and lowering cortisol levels, you can help heal the gut, improve digestive function, and restore the balance necessary for optimal health.

Environmental Toxins: The Role of Environmental Pollutants, Pesticides, and Endocrine Disruptors on Gut Health

Environmental toxins are everywhere. From the air we breathe to the food we consume, from household cleaning products to personal care items, exposure to harmful chemicals is a part of daily life. While many people focus on the immediate effects of pollutants and chemicals—such as respiratory issues, skin irritation, or cancer—few realize the profound impact these environmental toxins can have on our **gut health**.

The gut, often referred to as the body's "second brain," is highly sensitive to environmental stressors. An imbalance in gut health can lead to numerous health problems, ranging from digestive issues to autoimmune diseases and hormonal imbalances. In this section, we will delve into the specific role that **environmental pollutants, pesticides,** and **endocrine disruptors** play in damaging the gut lining, disrupting gut microbiota, and ultimately contributing to **leaky gut syndrome.**

1. What Are Environmental Toxins?

Environmental toxins are harmful substances that can contaminate the air, water, food, soil, and products that we come into contact with daily. These substances are often the result of human industrial activity and agriculture but can also be naturally occurring. They are typically classified into several categories:

- **Air pollutants**: These include **particulate matter, carbon monoxide, nitrogen dioxide**, and other airborne chemicals.
- **Water contaminants**: Pollutants like **heavy metals** (e.g., lead, mercury), **chlorine**, and **pharmaceuticals** found in water supplies.
- **Chemical residues**: Pesticides, herbicides, and fungicides used in agriculture, as well as preservatives and synthetic additives in processed food.
- **Endocrine disruptors**: Chemicals that interfere with the hormonal system, such as **bisphenol A (BPA), phthalates**, and **dioxins**.

Although environmental toxins vary widely, their collective impact on human health—especially gut health—can be devastating, and their role in exacerbating conditions like **leaky gut** is often underestimated.

2. The Gut as a Target for Environmental Toxins

The gut is a critical barrier that prevents harmful substances from entering the bloodstream, and it houses an intricate system of **immune cells, epithelial cells**, and **microorganisms** that work together to maintain homeostasis. However, the **gut lining** is highly susceptible to damage from environmental toxins, and prolonged exposure can compromise its integrity.

Gut Barrier Disruption

Environmental toxins, particularly those found in pesticides, herbicides, and industrial pollutants, can damage the **intestinal**

epithelial cells that form the gut lining. This damage weakens the **tight junctions**, the proteins that hold the cells together, leading to an increase in **intestinal permeability**, or **leaky gut**.

- **Pesticides**: Chemicals like **glyphosate** (the active ingredient in Roundup) are commonly used in agriculture but have been shown to disrupt the tight junctions in the gut. This can lead to a phenomenon known as **gut dysbiosis**, which occurs when the balance of gut bacteria is disrupted, promoting the growth of harmful bacteria and pathogens.
- **Heavy Metals**: Exposure to **heavy metals**, such as **mercury**, **cadmium**, and **lead**, can cause oxidative stress in the gut and disrupt the balance of gut microbiota. This promotes inflammation and damages the gut lining, further contributing to leaky gut.

Toxic Load and Inflammation

The gut is home to a large portion of the body's **immune system**, with **gut-associated lymphoid tissue (GALT)** playing a major role in immune defense. When environmental toxins breach the gut barrier and enter the bloodstream, they can trigger an **immune response**, leading to systemic **inflammation**. This chronic inflammation is one of the main contributors to **leaky gut** and many other autoimmune and chronic conditions.

- **Inflammation and Leaky Gut**: Persistent exposure to environmental toxins increases the production of **pro-inflammatory cytokines** that damage the intestinal lining and impair its ability to function properly. This perpetuates a cycle of inflammation and gut permeability, allowing harmful substances to leak into the bloodstream, further triggering the immune system and causing widespread systemic inflammation.

Impact on Gut Microbiota

The microbiome, the community of trillions of microorganisms that inhabit the gut, plays a critical role in digestion, immune function, and overall health. Environmental toxins can drastically affect the composition of the gut microbiota, promoting the growth of harmful bacteria and fungi while reducing beneficial species.

- **Glyphosate and Gut Dysbiosis**: Studies have shown that **glyphosate**, a commonly used pesticide, can alter the composition of gut bacteria, leading to **dysbiosis**—an imbalance of the gut microbiota. This imbalance can result in reduced diversity of beneficial bacteria, impairing the gut's ability to protect against harmful pathogens and contributing to **intestinal permeability**.
- **Antibiotics in Agriculture**: The use of antibiotics in agriculture to promote animal growth and prevent disease can also contribute to microbiome disruption. These antibiotics can pass through the food chain and impact the microbiota in humans, further damaging the gut ecosystem and making it more susceptible to **leaky gut**.

3. Endocrine Disruptors and Hormonal Imbalances in Women

Endocrine disruptors are chemicals that interfere with the **endocrine system**, which regulates the body's hormones. For women, who are especially sensitive to hormonal fluctuations throughout their lifetime, these chemicals can significantly disrupt hormonal balance and contribute to conditions like **estrogen dominance, PCOS**, and **menopausal symptoms**—all of which can impact gut health.

How Endocrine Disruptors Affect Gut Health

Many environmental toxins are known **endocrine disruptors**, including chemicals like **bisphenol A (BPA), phthalates**, and **polychlorinated biphenyls (PCBs)**. These substances can mimic or block hormones like estrogen and thyroid hormones, causing hormonal imbalances that negatively affect gut health.

- **Estrogen and Gut Permeability**: **Estrogen dominance**, a condition where there is an excess of estrogen relative to progesterone, can lead to increased intestinal permeability. Endocrine disruptors like BPA have been shown to increase estrogenic activity in the body, which may exacerbate gut permeability and contribute to leaky gut symptoms in women.
- **Thyroid Disruption**: Thyroid hormones play a role in maintaining gut motility and proper digestion. Environmental pollutants, especially **phthalates** and **polychlorinated**

biphenyls (PCBs), have been linked to thyroid dysfunction, which can further impair gut health. Thyroid imbalances can lead to **slower digestion**, constipation, and the **overgrowth of harmful bacteria**, all of which contribute to leaky gut.

Toxins and Menstrual Health

Environmental toxins can also affect **menstrual health** by disrupting the delicate balance of hormones like **estrogen** and **progesterone**. Hormonal fluctuations can lead to irregular periods, heavy bleeding, and increased risk of conditions like **fibroids** and **endometriosis**, all of which can have secondary effects on gut health.

- **Gut-Hormone Connection**: Hormones like estrogen influence the gut microbiome, and any disruption to these hormones can result in altered gut bacteria. For example, higher levels of estrogen during the luteal phase of the menstrual cycle can increase gut permeability, leading to exacerbated symptoms of **bloating**, **cramps**, and digestive discomfort.

4. Detoxifying from Environmental Toxins

Given the pervasive presence of environmental toxins in modern life, it's important to take steps to support the body's natural detoxification processes and reduce exposure to harmful chemicals. Here are a few strategies for reducing environmental toxin exposure and supporting gut health:

1. Avoiding Pesticides and Herbicides

- **Choose organic**: Whenever possible, opt for **organic** fruits and vegetables, which are grown without the use of harmful pesticides and herbicides like glyphosate.
- **Wash produce**: Thoroughly wash non-organic produce to reduce pesticide residues. Use a fruit and vegetable wash or a mixture of water and vinegar to remove chemicals from the surface.

2. Reducing Exposure to Endocrine Disruptors

- **Avoid BPA-containing plastics**: BPA (bisphenol A) is found in many plastic containers, food cans, and receipts. Use **BPA-free** plastics or switch to glass, stainless steel, or ceramic containers.

- **Choose natural personal care products**: Many personal care items, including shampoos, lotions, and cosmetics, contain **phthalates** and other endocrine-disrupting chemicals. Opt for products labeled as **paraben-free, phthalate-free**, and **organic**.

3. **Supporting Detoxification Pathways**
   - **Liver detox**: Support liver function by eating **liver-supportive foods** like cruciferous vegetables (broccoli, kale, cabbage), garlic, onions, and beets, which help the body process and eliminate toxins.
   - **Stay hydrated**: Drinking plenty of water helps flush toxins from the body and supports **kidney function** in detoxification.
   - **Increase fiber intake**: Fiber-rich foods such as whole grains, legumes, fruits, and vegetables help to cleanse the intestines and support regular bowel movements, which is essential for detoxifying the body.

Chapter 4: Leaky Gut and Women's Health Conditions: The Hidden Link

Leaky gut syndrome, or **intestinal permeability**, is increasingly recognized as a contributing factor to a wide range of health issues, particularly in women. While it's often dismissed as a vague or secondary health concern, the reality is that leaky gut is intricately linked to many conditions that disproportionately affect women. From **autoimmune diseases** to **hormonal imbalances** and **mental health disorders**, the impact of leaky gut on women's health is far-reaching.

In this chapter, we'll explore how leaky gut is connected to several women's health conditions, including **polycystic ovary syndrome (PCOS), endometriosis, autoimmune diseases**, and **mental health disorders**. We'll uncover the mechanisms that link gut health to these conditions, the role of systemic inflammation, and how addressing leaky gut can be a foundational step in improving overall health.

1. Leaky Gut and Autoimmune Diseases in Women

Women are significantly more likely than men to develop **autoimmune diseases**, which occur when the immune system mistakenly attacks the body's own tissues. Conditions like **Hashimoto's thyroiditis, lupus, rheumatoid arthritis**, and **multiple sclerosis** are far more prevalent in women, and emerging research suggests that **leaky**

gut may play a pivotal role in their development.

The Role of Gut Permeability in Autoimmune Disorders

The gut is home to the majority of the body's immune cells, making it a critical component of immune regulation. When the intestinal barrier becomes compromised, toxins, pathogens, and undigested food particles can enter the bloodstream, triggering an **immune response**. Over time, this constant activation of the immune system can lead to **chronic inflammation** and the development of autoimmune diseases.

- **Molecular Mimicry**: A key mechanism linking leaky gut to autoimmunity is **molecular mimicry**, where the immune system confuses its own tissues with foreign invaders. For example, bacterial proteins that leak into the bloodstream may resemble thyroid proteins, prompting the immune system to attack the thyroid gland, leading to conditions like **Hashimoto's thyroiditis**.
- **Increased Inflammation**: Chronic gut permeability leads to the release of pro-inflammatory cytokines, which further exacerbate autoimmune symptoms and damage tissues.

Autoimmune Conditions Linked to Leaky Gut

- **Hashimoto's Thyroiditis**: The most common cause of hypothyroidism in women, this autoimmune condition has been strongly associated with gut health. Addressing leaky gut can reduce inflammation and improve thyroid function.
- **Rheumatoid Arthritis**: Joint inflammation and pain in RA may be triggered or worsened by leaky gut, as the immune system attacks proteins in the joints due to systemic inflammation originating in the gut.
- **Lupus**: Women with lupus often experience gut inflammation and dysbiosis, which are closely tied to the progression of the disease.

2. Hormonal Imbalances and Leaky Gut

Women's hormonal cycles—regulated by **estrogen, progesterone,** and other key hormones—are sensitive to disruptions in gut health. Leaky gut can worsen hormonal imbalances, leading to or exacerbating conditions like **polycystic ovary syndrome (PCOS)**, endometriosis, and **estrogen dominance**.

Estrogen and Gut Health

The gut plays a crucial role in regulating estrogen levels through the **estrobolome**, a subset of gut bacteria that metabolizes and excretes estrogen. When the gut is imbalanced due to leaky gut, estrogen metabolism is disrupted, leading to **estrogen dominance**. This imbalance can exacerbate conditions such as **endometriosis** and **PMS**.

- **Endometriosis**: In women with endometriosis, chronic inflammation caused by leaky gut can worsen symptoms like pelvic pain and heavy menstrual bleeding. Additionally, disrupted estrogen metabolism further fuels the growth of endometrial tissue outside the uterus.
- **PCOS**: Women with PCOS often have increased gut inflammation and insulin resistance, both of which can be linked to leaky gut. Healing the gut may help reduce systemic inflammation and improve hormonal balance.

Cortisol and Stress

Chronic stress and elevated cortisol levels, which are common among women balancing work, family, and other demands, can weaken the gut lining and contribute to hormonal imbalances. Leaky gut perpetuates this cycle by increasing cortisol production through systemic inflammation, further disrupting hormones.

3. Mental Health and the Gut-Brain Axis

Women are nearly twice as likely as men to experience **anxiety**, **depression**, and other mood disorders. The connection between leaky gut and mental health lies in the **gut-brain axis**, a bi-directional communication network linking the gut and brain through the vagus nerve, immune system, and hormonal pathways.

How Leaky Gut Affects Mental Health

- **Chronic Inflammation**: When the gut is permeable, inflammatory cytokines can cross the blood-brain barrier, triggering neuroinflammation. This inflammation has been linked to symptoms of anxiety, depression, and cognitive dysfunction.
- **Neurotransmitter Production**: The gut produces a significant

amount of the body's serotonin, the "feel-good" neurotransmitter. A compromised gut can reduce serotonin production, contributing to mood disorders.
- **Brain Fog**: Many women with leaky gut report difficulty concentrating, memory lapses, and mental fatigue, collectively referred to as **brain fog**. This may be due to inflammation and the effects of dysbiosis on neurotransmitter balance.

Conditions Impacted by Leaky Gut

- **Postpartum Depression**: The stress of childbirth, hormonal shifts, and changes to the microbiome during pregnancy can increase gut permeability, potentially contributing to postpartum depression.
- **Premenstrual Dysphoric Disorder (PMDD)**: Women with PMDD often experience mood swings and heightened anxiety before their periods, which may be linked to gut-related inflammation and disrupted estrogen metabolism.

4. Skin Conditions and Leaky Gut

The phrase "you are what you eat" is particularly true for women's skin health. Skin conditions like **acne, rosacea, eczema**, and **psoriasis** are frequently tied to gut health, with leaky gut being a hidden driver of chronic skin inflammation.

Gut-Skin Axis

The gut-skin axis describes the connection between gut health and skin health. When the gut is leaky, it allows toxins and inflammatory compounds to enter the bloodstream, which can lead to skin flare-ups.

- **Acne**: Inflammation caused by leaky gut can stimulate sebaceous glands, leading to clogged pores and acne breakouts.
- **Eczema and Psoriasis**: These inflammatory skin conditions are often linked to autoimmune activity, which can be exacerbated by leaky gut. Healing the gut can reduce systemic inflammation and improve skin symptoms.

5. Digestive Disorders and Leaky Gut

Women are more likely to experience digestive disorders like **irritable bowel syndrome (IBS)** and **inflammatory bowel disease (IBD)**, both of which are closely linked to leaky gut.

IBS and Leaky Gut

IBS is characterized by symptoms like bloating, abdominal pain, and irregular bowel movements. While the exact cause of IBS is unknown, research shows that leaky gut and gut dysbiosis play significant roles in its development.

- **Gut Permeability and Symptoms**: Increased intestinal permeability allows substances to irritate the gut lining, triggering the abdominal pain and bloating associated with IBS.

IBD and Autoimmunity

Inflammatory bowel diseases like **Crohn's disease** and **ulcerative colitis** involve chronic inflammation of the digestive tract. Leaky gut can worsen inflammation and exacerbate symptoms like diarrhea, weight loss, and malnutrition.

PCOS, Endometriosis, and Leaky Gut: The Connection Between These Common Women's Health Conditions and Leaky Gut

Polycystic ovary syndrome (PCOS) and endometriosis are two of the most prevalent and challenging gynecological conditions affecting women's health today. These conditions are complex, involving hormonal imbalances, inflammation, and systemic health disruptions. Emerging research has highlighted the role of **leaky gut syndrome** in exacerbating these conditions, creating a critical link between gut health and women's reproductive health. Understanding this connection is essential for managing symptoms and improving overall well-being.

In this section, we will explore how **leaky gut** contributes to the development and progression of **PCOS** and **endometriosis**, the shared mechanisms linking these conditions, and strategies to address gut health as part of a holistic treatment approach.

1. PCOS and Leaky Gut

Polycystic ovary syndrome (PCOS) affects an estimated 1 in 10 women of reproductive age and is characterized by **hormonal imbalances, insulin resistance**, and the presence of **cysts on the ovaries**. While the exact cause of PCOS is unknown, inflammation and metabolic dysfunction play central roles in its development—and leaky gut may be a driving factor.

How Leaky Gut Contributes to PCOS
1. **Systemic Inflammation**
   - In women with PCOS, chronic inflammation is a hallmark symptom. **Leaky gut** exacerbates this by allowing toxins, bacteria, and undigested food particles to pass into the bloodstream, triggering an immune response. This immune activation leads to the release of **pro-inflammatory cytokines**, which worsen insulin resistance and hormonal imbalances.
   - **Cytokine Storm**: Elevated inflammatory cytokines like **TNF-alpha** and **IL-6** can disrupt ovarian function, impairing egg quality and contributing to irregular menstrual cycles.
2. **Insulin Resistance**
   - Insulin resistance is a defining feature of PCOS, and leaky gut can worsen this condition. When the gut barrier is compromised, it allows **lipopolysaccharides (LPS)**—inflammatory molecules from gut bacteria—to enter the bloodstream. LPS has been shown to impair insulin signaling, exacerbating insulin resistance and contributing to weight gain, a common symptom in women with PCOS.
   - **Gut Dysbiosis**: Imbalances in gut bacteria caused by leaky gut can also alter metabolism and energy regulation, further contributing to weight challenges and insulin resistance.
3. **Gut-Hormone Axis**
   - The **gut microbiota** plays a crucial role in regulating estrogen levels through the **estrobolome**, a subset of bacteria involved in estrogen metabolism. In women with PCOS, disrupted gut bacteria caused by leaky gut can impair estrogen regulation, contributing to symptoms like **hirsutism, acne**, and irregular cycles.

2. Endometriosis and Leaky Gut
Endometriosis is a chronic condition where **endometrial-like tissue**

grows outside the uterus, causing severe pain, inflammation, and, in some cases, infertility. Although the exact cause of endometriosis remains unclear, research has increasingly pointed to the role of **chronic inflammation** and **immune dysfunction**—both of which are exacerbated by leaky gut.

How Leaky Gut Contributes to Endometriosis

1. **Chronic Inflammation**
   - Women with endometriosis often experience heightened **systemic inflammation,** which worsens symptoms like pelvic pain, bloating, and fatigue. Leaky gut perpetuates this inflammation by allowing harmful substances to leak into the bloodstream, activating the immune system and increasing the production of inflammatory mediators like **prostaglandins** and **cytokines.**
   - **Inflammation and Adhesions**: Chronic inflammation can also promote the formation of adhesions and scar tissue, a hallmark of endometriosis.

2. **Immune Dysregulation**
   - The immune system plays a significant role in the progression of endometriosis. Leaky gut compromises the gut-associated lymphoid tissue (**GALT**), which houses a large portion of the body's immune cells. This dysregulation weakens the body's ability to clear misplaced endometrial tissue and may contribute to the condition's progression.

3. **Estrogen Dominance**
   - Endometriosis is an estrogen-driven condition, and leaky gut can exacerbate **estrogen dominance**. A disrupted gut microbiota affects the body's ability to metabolize and excrete estrogen, leading to higher circulating levels of this hormone. Elevated estrogen fuels the growth of endometrial tissue, worsening symptoms.

4. **Pain Sensitization**
   - The inflammatory cytokines released due to leaky gut can sensitize nerves, worsening the **chronic pelvic pain** that

is characteristic of endometriosis. This connection highlights the importance of addressing gut inflammation to manage pain effectively.

3. Shared Mechanisms: The Gut-Hormone-Immune Triad

Both PCOS and endometriosis share common underlying mechanisms that are directly influenced by leaky gut. These include:

1. Inflammation
- In both conditions, chronic inflammation is a driving force behind symptoms and disease progression. Leaky gut amplifies systemic inflammation, creating a vicious cycle that worsens hormonal imbalances and immune dysfunction.

2. Hormonal Disruption
- The **gut microbiota** plays a central role in metabolizing and regulating hormones like estrogen and progesterone. Leaky gut disrupts this process, contributing to hormonal imbalances that drive PCOS and endometriosis.

3. Immune System Dysregulation
- Leaky gut impairs the immune system's ability to distinguish between harmful invaders and the body's own tissues, a phenomenon that contributes to autoimmune-like reactions in both conditions.

4. Gut Dysbiosis
- An imbalance in gut bacteria is common in women with PCOS and endometriosis. Dysbiosis caused by leaky gut further disrupts digestion, hormone regulation, and immune function, exacerbating symptoms.

4. Healing the Gut to Address PCOS and Endometriosis

Given the strong connection between leaky gut, PCOS, and endometriosis, addressing gut health can be a powerful strategy for managing symptoms and improving overall health. Here are key strategies to heal the gut and support hormonal balance:

1. Anti-Inflammatory Diet
- Focus on foods that reduce inflammation and promote gut healing, such as:
  - **Fruits and vegetables**: High in antioxidants and fiber.

- **Omega-3 fatty acids**: Found in fatty fish, flaxseeds, and walnuts.
- **Fermented foods**: Yogurt, kefir, sauerkraut, and kimchi support the growth of beneficial gut bacteria.

2. Avoid Trigger Foods
- Eliminate foods that worsen gut inflammation, including:
  - Gluten
  - Dairy
  - Refined sugar
  - Processed foods
- An **elimination diet** can help identify specific food sensitivities.

3. Support Gut Microbiota
- Take **probiotics** to restore balance to the gut microbiome.
- Include **prebiotic fibers** like those found in bananas, garlic, and asparagus to feed beneficial bacteria.

4. Reduce Toxin Exposure
- Limit exposure to **environmental toxins** such as pesticides and endocrine disruptors, which can worsen leaky gut and hormonal imbalances.

5. Manage Stress
- Chronic stress increases **cortisol levels**, which can weaken the gut lining and exacerbate symptoms. Incorporate stress-reducing activities such as yoga, meditation, or regular exercise.

6. Supplement Wisely
- **L-glutamine**: Supports gut lining repair.
- **Vitamin D**: Helps modulate the immune system and reduce inflammation.
- **Magnesium**: Can help regulate hormonal imbalances and reduce inflammation.

Gut Health and Menstrual Cycle: How Your Gut Influences Menstrual Health, Including Mood Swings, Cramps, and Bloating

The **gut** and the **menstrual cycle** are intricately connected through a complex web of hormonal, inflammatory, and microbial pathways. While the menstrual cycle is primarily governed by hormones like **estrogen**, **progesterone**, and **prostaglandins**, the gut microbiome plays a significant role in modulating these hormones and influencing menstrual health. For many women, symptoms like **mood swings, cramps**, and **bloating** during their menstrual cycle may stem not just from hormonal fluctuations but also from underlying issues in gut health.

In this section, we will explore the **gut-menstrual connection**, uncover how the gut microbiome and intestinal health influence menstrual symptoms, and provide actionable strategies to optimize gut health for better menstrual well-being.

1. The Gut-Hormone Connection: Regulating Menstrual Health

The gut and hormones are in constant communication through the **gut-hormone axis**, where the gut microbiome and intestinal function directly influence the production, metabolism, and regulation of key hormones involved in the menstrual cycle.

The Role of the Gut Microbiome

The gut microbiome, a diverse ecosystem of bacteria, viruses, and fungi residing in the digestive tract, is essential for maintaining hormonal balance. A healthy and balanced microbiome supports proper digestion, immune function, and the regulation of **estrogen** and **progesterone**.

- **The Estrobolome**: A subset of gut bacteria known as the **estrobolome** is responsible for metabolizing estrogen and regulating its levels in the body. The estrobolome produces enzymes that break down estrogen in the liver, allowing it to be excreted through the digestive system. If the gut microbiome is imbalanced (a condition known as **dysbiosis**), estrogen metabolism can be disrupted, leading to **estrogen dominance**—a common contributor to menstrual symptoms like bloating, heavy periods, and mood swings.

How Gut Health Affects Hormonal Balance

1. **Estrogen Regulation:**
    - An imbalanced microbiome can impair estrogen detoxification, resulting in higher levels of circulating estrogen. This can exacerbate symptoms like PMS, breast tenderness, and painful cramps.
    - Conversely, insufficient estrogen clearance can affect ovulation, leading to irregular or missed periods.

2. **Progesterone and Gut Health**:
   - Progesterone, which rises during the second half of the menstrual cycle, has a calming effect on the gut, promoting smooth digestion. However, low progesterone levels can lead to **constipation** or **sluggish digestion**, which may worsen bloating and discomfort.
3. **Cortisol and Stress**:
   - Chronic stress and elevated cortisol levels disrupt the gut lining, contributing to **leaky gut syndrome** and systemic inflammation. High cortisol also suppresses progesterone production, creating a hormonal imbalance that worsens PMS symptoms.

2. Gut Health and Common Menstrual Symptoms

The health of your gut influences the severity and frequency of many menstrual symptoms, including **mood swings, cramps,** and **bloating**. Here's how:

Mood Swings and the Gut-Brain Axis

The **gut-brain axis** is the communication network between the gut and the brain, facilitated by the vagus nerve, neurotransmitters, and the immune system. The gut microbiome plays a critical role in producing **neurotransmitters** that regulate mood, including **serotonin, dopamine,** and **GABA**.

- **Serotonin Production**: Approximately 90% of the body's serotonin, the "feel-good" neurotransmitter, is produced in the gut. When the gut microbiome is imbalanced, serotonin production can be impaired, contributing to **mood swings, anxiety,** and **depression** during the menstrual cycle.
- **Inflammation and Mood**: Dysbiosis and leaky gut can lead to the release of pro-inflammatory cytokines, which cross the blood-brain barrier and contribute to symptoms like irritability and brain fog.

Menstrual Cramps and Gut Inflammation

Menstrual cramps, or **dysmenorrhea**, are caused by the release of **prostaglandins**, hormone-like substances that trigger uterine contractions. Gut health plays a role in modulating inflammation, which

can either worsen or alleviate the severity of cramps.
- **Prostaglandin Production**: An inflamed gut can increase the production of inflammatory prostaglandins, worsening the intensity of cramps.
- **Magnesium and Cramp Relief**: A healthy gut microbiome aids in the absorption of **magnesium**, a mineral that helps relax muscles and reduce cramps. Poor gut health can impair magnesium absorption, exacerbating menstrual pain.

Bloating and Gut Function

Bloating is one of the most common menstrual symptoms and is closely tied to gut health.
- **Estrogen and Water Retention**: High estrogen levels during the menstrual cycle can lead to water retention and bloating. An imbalanced gut microbiome can impair estrogen clearance, exacerbating this symptom.
- **Gas and Dysbiosis**: Gut dysbiosis can lead to **excessive gas production**, which contributes to bloating and abdominal discomfort. Additionally, hormonal fluctuations during the luteal phase can slow digestion, further increasing bloating.

3. How the Menstrual Cycle Impacts Gut Health

Just as gut health influences the menstrual cycle, hormonal fluctuations during the menstrual cycle also affect the gut. Women often experience changes in digestion, appetite, and gut motility at different phases of their cycle.

Follicular Phase (Day 1–14)

- **Estrogen Rise**: During this phase, estrogen levels gradually increase, promoting healthy gut motility and microbial diversity. Women often experience fewer digestive issues in this phase.

Luteal Phase (Day 15–28)

- **Progesterone and Slow Digestion**: Progesterone peaks during the luteal phase, slowing gut motility and leading to symptoms like constipation and bloating. Gut inflammation and dysbiosis can worsen these symptoms.
- **Cravings and Gut Microbiota**: Hormonal shifts during the luteal phase can lead to cravings for sugary or high-carb foods,

which feed harmful gut bacteria and exacerbate dysbiosis.

Menstrual Phase (Day 1–7 of Next Cycle)
- **Prostaglandin Surge**: The release of prostaglandins during menstruation can increase inflammation and exacerbate symptoms like cramps and diarrhea, especially if gut health is compromised.

4. Optimizing Gut Health for Better Menstrual Health

Improving gut health can significantly reduce menstrual symptoms like mood swings, cramps, and bloating. Here are actionable strategies to support gut health throughout your menstrual cycle:

1. Anti-Inflammatory Diet
- **Eat Whole Foods**: Focus on nutrient-dense foods like leafy greens, berries, fatty fish, nuts, and seeds that reduce inflammation.
- **Avoid Processed Foods**: Minimize sugar, refined carbs, and artificial additives, which can disrupt gut bacteria.

2. Support Gut Microbiota
- **Probiotics**: Incorporate probiotic-rich foods like yogurt, kefir, sauerkraut, and kimchi to boost beneficial bacteria.
- **Prebiotics**: Feed your gut bacteria with prebiotic foods like bananas, garlic, onions, and asparagus.

3. Balance Hormones
- **Fiber-Rich Foods**: Fiber aids in the elimination of excess estrogen. Include flaxseeds, chia seeds, and vegetables in your diet.
- **Healthy Fats**: Omega-3 fatty acids, found in salmon and walnuts, support hormonal balance and reduce inflammation.

4. Manage Stress
- Practice **mindfulness, meditation,** and **yoga** to reduce stress and cortisol levels, which impact gut and hormonal health.

5. Stay Hydrated
- Drink plenty of water to support digestion and reduce bloating during your cycle.

6. Address Specific Deficiencies
- **Magnesium**: Supplement magnesium to relieve cramps and

support gut health.
- **Vitamin B6**: Helps regulate mood and reduce PMS symptoms.
- **Zinc**: Supports gut healing and reduces inflammation.

Gut Health and Menstrual Cycle: How Your Gut Influences Menstrual Health, Including Mood Swings, Cramps, and Bloating

The **gut** and the **menstrual cycle** are intricately connected through a complex web of hormonal, inflammatory, and microbial pathways. While the menstrual cycle is primarily governed by hormones like **estrogen**, **progesterone**, and **prostaglandins**, the gut microbiome plays a significant role in modulating these hormones and influencing menstrual health. For many women, symptoms like **mood swings**, **cramps**, and **bloating** during their menstrual cycle may stem not just from hormonal fluctuations but also from underlying issues in gut health.

In this section, we will explore the **gut-menstrual connection**, uncover how the gut microbiome and intestinal health influence menstrual symptoms, and provide actionable strategies to optimize gut health for better menstrual well-being.

1. The Gut-Hormone Connection: Regulating Menstrual Health

The gut and hormones are in constant communication through the **gut-hormone axis**, where the gut microbiome and intestinal function directly influence the production, metabolism, and regulation of key hormones involved in the menstrual cycle.

The Role of the Gut Microbiome

The gut microbiome, a diverse ecosystem of bacteria, viruses, and fungi residing in the digestive tract, is essential for maintaining hormonal balance. A healthy and balanced microbiome supports proper digestion, immune function, and the regulation of **estrogen** and **progesterone**.

- **The Estrobolome**: A subset of gut bacteria known as the **estrobolome** is responsible for metabolizing estrogen and regulating its levels in the body. The estrobolome produces enzymes that break down estrogen in the liver, allowing it to be excreted through the digestive system. If the gut microbiome is imbalanced (a condition known as **dysbiosis**), estrogen metabolism can be disrupted, leading to **estrogen dominance**—a common contributor to menstrual symptoms like bloating, heavy periods, and mood swings.

How Gut Health Affects Hormonal Balance

1. **Estrogen Regulation**:
   - An imbalanced microbiome can impair estrogen detoxification, resulting in higher levels of circulating estrogen. This can exacerbate symptoms like PMS, breast tenderness, and painful cramps.
   - Conversely, insufficient estrogen clearance can affect ovulation, leading to irregular or missed periods.
2. **Progesterone and Gut Health**:
   - Progesterone, which rises during the second half of the menstrual cycle, has a calming effect on the gut, promoting smooth digestion. However, low progesterone levels can lead to **constipation** or **sluggish digestion**, which may worsen bloating and discomfort.
3. **Cortisol and Stress**:
   - Chronic stress and elevated cortisol levels disrupt the gut lining, contributing to **leaky gut syndrome** and systemic inflammation. High cortisol also suppresses progesterone production, creating a hormonal imbalance that worsens PMS symptoms.

2. Gut Health and Common Menstrual Symptoms

The health of your gut influences the severity and frequency of many menstrual symptoms, including **mood swings, cramps,** and **bloating**. Here's how:

Mood Swings and the Gut-Brain Axis

The **gut-brain axis** is the communication network between the gut and the brain, facilitated by the vagus nerve, neurotransmitters, and the immune system. The gut microbiome plays a critical role in producing **neurotransmitters** that regulate mood, including **serotonin, dopamine,** and **GABA**.

- **Serotonin Production**: Approximately 90% of the body's serotonin, the "feel-good" neurotransmitter, is produced in the gut. When the gut microbiome is imbalanced, serotonin production can be impaired, contributing to **mood swings,**

anxiety, and **depression** during the menstrual cycle.
- **Inflammation and Mood**: Dysbiosis and leaky gut can lead to the release of pro-inflammatory cytokines, which cross the blood-brain barrier and contribute to symptoms like irritability and brain fog.

Menstrual Cramps and Gut Inflammation

Menstrual cramps, or **dysmenorrhea**, are caused by the release of **prostaglandins**, hormone-like substances that trigger uterine contractions. Gut health plays a role in modulating inflammation, which can either worsen or alleviate the severity of cramps.
- **Prostaglandin Production**: An inflamed gut can increase the production of inflammatory prostaglandins, worsening the intensity of cramps.
- **Magnesium and Cramp Relief**: A healthy gut microbiome aids in the absorption of **magnesium**, a mineral that helps relax muscles and reduce cramps. Poor gut health can impair magnesium absorption, exacerbating menstrual pain.

Bloating and Gut Function

Bloating is one of the most common menstrual symptoms and is closely tied to gut health.
- **Estrogen and Water Retention**: High estrogen levels during the menstrual cycle can lead to water retention and bloating. An imbalanced gut microbiome can impair estrogen clearance, exacerbating this symptom.
- **Gas and Dysbiosis**: Gut dysbiosis can lead to **excessive gas production**, which contributes to bloating and abdominal discomfort. Additionally, hormonal fluctuations during the luteal phase can slow digestion, further increasing bloating.

3. How the Menstrual Cycle Impacts Gut Health

Just as gut health influences the menstrual cycle, hormonal fluctuations during the menstrual cycle also affect the gut. Women often experience changes in digestion, appetite, and gut motility at different phases of their cycle.

Follicular Phase (Day 1–14)
- **Estrogen Rise**: During this phase, estrogen levels gradually

increase, promoting healthy gut motility and microbial diversity. Women often experience fewer digestive issues in this phase.

Luteal Phase (Day 15–28)
- **Progesterone and Slow Digestion**: Progesterone peaks during the luteal phase, slowing gut motility and leading to symptoms like constipation and bloating. Gut inflammation and dysbiosis can worsen these symptoms.
- **Cravings and Gut Microbiota**: Hormonal shifts during the luteal phase can lead to cravings for sugary or high-carb foods, which feed harmful gut bacteria and exacerbate dysbiosis.

Menstrual Phase (Day 1–7 of Next Cycle)
- **Prostaglandin Surge**: The release of prostaglandins during menstruation can increase inflammation and exacerbate symptoms like cramps and diarrhea, especially if gut health is compromised.

4. Optimizing Gut Health for Better Menstrual Health

Improving gut health can significantly reduce menstrual symptoms like mood swings, cramps, and bloating. Here are actionable strategies to support gut health throughout your menstrual cycle:

1. Anti-Inflammatory Diet
- **Eat Whole Foods**: Focus on nutrient-dense foods like leafy greens, berries, fatty fish, nuts, and seeds that reduce inflammation.
- **Avoid Processed Foods**: Minimize sugar, refined carbs, and artificial additives, which can disrupt gut bacteria.

2. Support Gut Microbiota
- **Probiotics**: Incorporate probiotic-rich foods like yogurt, kefir, sauerkraut, and kimchi to boost beneficial bacteria.
- **Prebiotics**: Feed your gut bacteria with prebiotic foods like bananas, garlic, onions, and asparagus.

3. Balance Hormones
- **Fiber-Rich Foods**: Fiber aids in the elimination of excess estrogen. Include flaxseeds, chia seeds, and vegetables in your diet.
- **Healthy Fats**: Omega-3 fatty acids, found in salmon and

walnuts, support hormonal balance and reduce inflammation.

4. Manage Stress
- Practice **mindfulness, meditation,** and **yoga** to reduce stress and cortisol levels, which impact gut and hormonal health.

5. Stay Hydrated
- Drink plenty of water to support digestion and reduce bloating during your cycle.

6. Address Specific Deficiencies
- **Magnesium**: Supplement magnesium to relieve cramps and support gut health.
- **Vitamin B6**: Helps regulate mood and reduce PMS symptoms.
- **Zinc**: Supports gut healing and reduces inflammation.

Thyroid and Leaky Gut: The Role of Gut Health in Thyroid Imbalances and Autoimmune Thyroid Conditions Like Hashimoto's

The **thyroid gland**, a small butterfly-shaped organ located in the neck, plays a critical role in regulating metabolism, energy production, and overall hormonal balance. However, thyroid imbalances, including **hypothyroidism** and **autoimmune thyroid conditions** like **Hashimoto's thyroiditis**, have become increasingly prevalent, particularly among women. While these conditions are often linked to genetic, hormonal, and environmental factors, recent research highlights the crucial role of **gut health** in the development and progression of thyroid disorders.

Leaky gut syndrome (or **intestinal permeability**) is emerging as a key contributor to thyroid imbalances, especially in autoimmune conditions like Hashimoto's. By disrupting the delicate balance of the immune system, gut microbiome, and intestinal barrier, leaky gut creates a cascade of inflammatory and autoimmune responses that directly impact thyroid function. In this chapter, we will explore the connection between gut health and thyroid conditions, focusing on the mechanisms linking leaky gut to thyroid dysfunction and practical steps to improve gut health for thyroid support.

1. The Gut-Thyroid Connection

The gut and thyroid are intricately linked through the **gut-thyroid**

axis, a bi-directional communication pathway where the health of the gut influences thyroid function and vice versa. The gut's role in thyroid health can be understood through several mechanisms:

a. Immune System Regulation
- Approximately **70% of the immune system** resides in the gut, in the form of **gut-associated lymphoid tissue (GALT)**. A healthy gut helps maintain immune tolerance, preventing the immune system from mistakenly attacking its own tissues. However, when the gut barrier is compromised (as in leaky gut), this immune balance is disrupted, increasing the risk of **autoimmune diseases** like Hashimoto's thyroiditis.

b. Thyroid Hormone Conversion
- The majority of **thyroxine (T4)**, the inactive thyroid hormone produced by the thyroid gland, is converted to its active form, **triiodothyronine (T3)**, in the liver and gut. A healthy gut microbiome supports this conversion process. Dysbiosis (an imbalance in gut bacteria) can impair T4-to-T3 conversion, contributing to hypothyroid symptoms like fatigue, weight gain, and brain fog.

c. Gut Microbiota and Hormonal Balance
- The gut microbiome plays a role in regulating hormone metabolism, including the clearance of **thyroid hormones**. Dysbiosis and leaky gut can slow down the metabolism and excretion of hormones, leading to imbalances that worsen thyroid function.

d. Chronic Inflammation
- Leaky gut leads to systemic **inflammation**, which directly impairs thyroid function. Inflammation increases levels of **reverse T3 (rT3)**, an inactive form of T3 that competes with active T3, reducing the body's ability to use thyroid hormones effectively.

2. Leaky Gut and Hashimoto's Thyroiditis

Hashimoto's thyroiditis is the most common autoimmune condition affecting the thyroid, particularly in women. It occurs when the immune system produces antibodies that attack the thyroid gland, leading to inflammation and eventual hypothyroidism. **Leaky gut** is a significant trigger and perpetuator of this condition.

How Leaky Gut Contributes to Hashimoto's

1. **Increased Intestinal Permeability**
   - In a healthy gut, tight junctions between intestinal cells act as a barrier, allowing only nutrients to pass into the bloodstream. In leaky gut syndrome, these tight junctions become compromised, allowing harmful substances like undigested food particles, toxins, and bacteria to "leak" into the bloodstream.
   - These substances are recognized as foreign invaders by the immune system, triggering chronic inflammation and increasing the likelihood of autoimmune responses, including the production of **thyroid autoantibodies** like **TPOAb** (thyroid peroxidase antibodies) and **TGAb** (thyroglobulin antibodies).

2. **Molecular Mimicry**
   - Certain proteins found in foods, bacteria, or viruses that enter the bloodstream through a leaky gut resemble thyroid tissue proteins. This phenomenon, known as **molecular mimicry**, causes the immune system to mistakenly attack the thyroid gland, perpetuating Hashimoto's thyroiditis.

3. **Gut Dysbiosis**
   - Dysbiosis, or an imbalance in the gut microbiome, is common in individuals with Hashimoto's. Harmful bacteria in the gut produce **lipopolysaccharides (LPS)**, inflammatory molecules that exacerbate gut permeability and systemic inflammation, fueling thyroid autoimmunity.

4. **Chronic Inflammation and Thyroid Damage**
   - Chronic low-grade inflammation caused by leaky gut increases the production of pro-inflammatory cytokines. These cytokines interfere with thyroid function by damaging thyroid cells and altering the production of

thyroid hormones.

3. Symptoms of Gut-Related Thyroid Dysfunction

The effects of leaky gut on thyroid health can manifest as a range of symptoms, many of which overlap with typical hypothyroid symptoms. These include:

- **Digestive Symptoms**: Bloating, gas, constipation, diarrhea, or irritable bowel syndrome (IBS).
- **Fatigue**: Persistent tiredness due to impaired thyroid hormone conversion and chronic inflammation.
- **Brain Fog**: Difficulty concentrating, poor memory, and mental fatigue caused by gut inflammation and reduced T3 levels.
- **Weight Gain**: Sluggish metabolism due to thyroid dysfunction and insulin resistance linked to gut dysbiosis.
- **Hair Loss and Dry Skin**: Reduced thyroid function impacts skin and hair health.
- **Joint Pain and Muscle Weakness**: Systemic inflammation from leaky gut contributes to musculoskeletal symptoms.
- **Mood Disturbances**: Anxiety and depression linked to gut dysbiosis and inflammation.

4. Supporting Gut Health to Improve Thyroid Function

Healing the gut is a foundational step in managing thyroid conditions like Hashimoto's and optimizing overall thyroid health. Here are actionable strategies to address leaky gut and support thyroid function:

a. Anti-Inflammatory Diet

Adopting an anti-inflammatory diet can help reduce gut inflammation and repair the intestinal lining.

- **Eliminate Trigger Foods**: Avoid gluten, dairy, refined sugar, soy, and processed foods, which can trigger inflammation and exacerbate leaky gut.
- **Include Gut-Healing Foods**:
  - **Bone broth**: Rich in collagen and amino acids like **L-glutamine**, which help repair the gut lining.
  - **Fermented foods**: Yogurt, kefir, sauerkraut, and kimchi to restore gut microbiota.
  - **High-fiber foods**: Vegetables, fruits, and legumes to

feed beneficial gut bacteria.

b. Reduce Toxin Exposure
- Avoid environmental toxins like pesticides, BPA, and phthalates, which can contribute to gut permeability and hormonal imbalances.

c. Supplement Wisely

Certain supplements can help heal the gut and support thyroid function:
- **Probiotics**: Restore balance in the gut microbiome and reduce inflammation.
- **L-glutamine**: Repairs the gut lining and supports intestinal barrier integrity.
- **Zinc and Selenium**: Essential for thyroid hormone production and immune regulation.
- **Vitamin D**: Modulates the immune system and reduces inflammation.

d. Manage Stress

Chronic stress increases cortisol levels, which can worsen leaky gut and impair thyroid function. Incorporate stress-reducing practices like:
- Yoga
- Meditation
- Deep breathing exercises

e. Address Gut Dysbiosis
- Work with a healthcare provider to address overgrowth of harmful bacteria, yeast (e.g., candida), or parasites through targeted antimicrobial or antifungal treatments.

5. The Importance of Testing for Gut and Thyroid Health

Identifying and addressing leaky gut and thyroid dysfunction requires proper testing. Some recommended tests include:
- **Thyroid Panel**: To check TSH, free T4, free T3, reverse T3, and thyroid antibodies (TPOAb and TGAb).
- **Comprehensive Stool Analysis**: To assess gut microbiota, inflammation markers, and digestive function.
- **Zonulin Levels**: A biomarker for intestinal permeability.
- **Food Sensitivity Testing**: To identify and eliminate

inflammatory foods that exacerbate leaky gut.

Chapter 5: Nutrition for Healing Leaky Gut: The Best Foods to Eat

Healing **leaky gut syndrome** begins with proper nutrition. The foods you consume can either harm or heal your gut lining, influence inflammation, and restore balance to your **gut microbiome**. By prioritizing **gut-friendly foods**, you can repair the intestinal barrier, reduce systemic inflammation, and alleviate symptoms of leaky gut and related health conditions.

In this chapter, we'll explore the **best foods to eat** for healing leaky gut, explaining their benefits and how they support gut health. We'll also provide practical tips for incorporating these foods into your daily diet for long-term success.

1. Understanding Gut-Healing Nutrition

To heal leaky gut, your diet should focus on three key principles:
1. **Reducing inflammation** in the gut lining.
2. **Rebuilding and repairing the intestinal barrier**.
3. **Restoring balance to the gut microbiome**.

The foods listed in this chapter are carefully chosen for their ability to address these goals by:

- Providing essential nutrients like **amino acids, vitamins**, and **minerals**.
- Supporting beneficial bacteria in the gut.
- Eliminating triggers that may exacerbate intestinal permeability.

2. The Best Foods to Heal Leaky Gut

a. Bone Broth

Bone broth is one of the most effective foods for repairing the gut lining. It is rich in **collagen, gelatin**, and **amino acids** like **L-glutamine**, which are critical for rebuilding the intestinal barrier.

- **Benefits**:
    - Collagen and gelatin help seal the gut lining and reduce intestinal permeability.
    - L-glutamine provides fuel for enterocytes (intestinal cells) and aids in repairing damaged tissue.
    - Contains anti-inflammatory compounds that soothe the digestive tract.
- **How to Use**:
    - Drink warm bone broth as a comforting beverage.
    - Use it as a base for soups, stews, and sauces.

b. Fermented Foods

Fermented foods are packed with **probiotics**, which help restore balance to the gut microbiome by increasing beneficial bacteria.

- **Examples**:
    - Yogurt (unsweetened and full-fat)
    - Kefir
    - Sauerkraut
    - Kimchi
    - Miso
    - Pickles (fermented without vinegar)
- **Benefits**:
    - Improve digestion and nutrient absorption.
    - Reduce gut inflammation by balancing gut bacteria.
    - Support the production of **short-chain fatty acids (SCFAs)**, which nourish the gut lining.
- **How to Use**:

- Add a serving of fermented foods to meals as a side dish or topping.
- Start with small amounts and gradually increase to avoid digestive discomfort.

c. High-Fiber Foods

Fiber acts as a **prebiotic**, feeding beneficial bacteria and promoting a healthy gut environment. Soluble fiber, in particular, helps soothe inflammation and regulate digestion.

- **Examples**:
    - Fruits: Berries, apples, pears, bananas (ripe)
    - Vegetables: Asparagus, artichokes, carrots, zucchini
    - Whole grains: Oats, quinoa, millet
    - Legumes: Lentils, chickpeas
- **Benefits**:
    - Supports the growth of good bacteria in the gut.
    - Helps produce SCFAs, which maintain gut barrier integrity.
    - Promotes regular bowel movements and reduces bloating.
- **How to Use**:
    - Incorporate a variety of fiber-rich foods into every meal.
    - Pair fiber with healthy fats and proteins to avoid blood sugar spikes.

d. Healthy Fats

Anti-inflammatory fats are essential for reducing gut inflammation and supporting the repair of the gut lining.

- **Examples**:
    - Omega-3-rich foods: Salmon, sardines, mackerel, flaxseeds, chia seeds, walnuts
    - Monounsaturated fats: Olive oil, avocados, almond butter
    - Coconut oil: Contains **medium-chain triglycerides (MCTs)**, which are easily digested and support gut health.
- **Benefits**:

- Reduce chronic inflammation and support the immune system.
- Provide energy for healing and repair.
- Support the absorption of fat-soluble vitamins (A, D, E, and K).
- **How to Use:**
    - Cook with olive oil or coconut oil.
    - Add chia or flaxseeds to smoothies, yogurt, or oatmeal.

e. Anti-Inflammatory Vegetables

Certain vegetables contain **antioxidants** and **phytonutrients** that fight inflammation and support gut healing.

- **Examples**:
    - Leafy greens: Spinach, kale, Swiss chard
    - Cruciferous vegetables: Broccoli, cauliflower, Brussels sprouts
    - Colorful veggies: Sweet potatoes, beets, bell peppers
- **Benefits**:
    - Provide essential nutrients like **vitamins A and C**, which support the gut lining.
    - Contain fiber and prebiotics for microbial balance.
    - Reduce oxidative stress in the digestive tract.
- **How to Use:**
    - Steam or sauté vegetables to preserve nutrients and aid digestion.
    - Incorporate a variety of colors into meals for a broad range of nutrients.

f. Gut-Healing Proteins

Proteins are essential for repairing tissue and rebuilding the gut lining.

- **Examples**:
    - Pasture-raised chicken and turkey
    - Wild-caught fish
    - Grass-fed beef
    - Eggs
    - Plant-based options: Tofu, tempeh
- **Benefits**:

- Provide amino acids like **L-glutamine** and **glycine**, which heal the gut lining.
- Support the growth and repair of intestinal cells.
- **How to Use:**
    - Choose high-quality, minimally processed protein sources.
    - Incorporate protein into every meal to stabilize blood sugar and support gut repair.

g. Herbs and Spices

Certain herbs and spices have natural **anti-inflammatory** and **antimicrobial** properties that promote gut health.

- **Examples:**
    - Turmeric (with black pepper for absorption)
    - Ginger
    - Garlic (cooked to reduce harshness)
    - Cinnamon
    - Oregano
- **Benefits:**
    - Reduce inflammation in the gut lining.
    - Support digestion and microbial balance.
    - Combat harmful bacteria without disturbing beneficial bacteria.
- **How to Use:**
    - Add fresh or ground spices to meals, teas, or smoothies.
    - Use turmeric and ginger in soups or stews for a warming, gut-healing boost.

h. Healing Beverages

Staying hydrated and choosing gut-supportive beverages can aid digestion and reduce inflammation.

- **Examples:**
    - Herbal teas: Peppermint, chamomile, ginger, dandelion
    - Aloe vera juice (unsweetened)
    - Coconut water (unsweetened)
- **Benefits:**
    - Soothe the digestive tract and reduce bloating.

- Provide hydration to support cellular repair.
- Promote regular bowel movements and detoxification.
- **How to Use**:
  - Sip on herbal teas throughout the day.
  - Drink aloe vera juice in moderation to soothe the gut lining.

3. Foods to Avoid While Healing Leaky Gut

Equally important as the foods you eat are the foods you should avoid. Certain foods can irritate the gut lining, increase inflammation, and exacerbate leaky gut.

a. Gluten
- Found in wheat, barley, and rye, gluten is known to increase intestinal permeability in sensitive individuals.

b. Dairy
- Many people with leaky gut are sensitive to lactose or casein, both of which can trigger inflammation.

c. Refined Sugar
- Sugar feeds harmful bacteria and yeast, contributing to dysbiosis and inflammation.

d. Processed Foods
- Artificial additives, preservatives, and trans fats can irritate the gut lining and disrupt microbial balance.

e. Alcohol
- Alcohol damages the intestinal lining and increases gut permeability.

4. Practical Tips for Healing Leaky Gut with Nutrition

1. **Plan Balanced Meals**:
   - Include protein, healthy fats, and fiber in every meal to support gut repair and stabilize blood sugar.
2. **Cook at Home**:
   - Preparing your meals ensures you avoid inflammatory ingredients and prioritize fresh, gut-healing foods.
3. **Introduce New Foods Gradually**:
   - If you're incorporating fermented foods or fiber, start with small amounts to avoid digestive discomfort.

4. **Stay Hydrated**:
   - Drink plenty of water throughout the day to support digestion and nutrient absorption.
5. **Listen to Your Body**:
   - Pay attention to how your body reacts to different foods and adjust your diet accordingly.

Gut-Healing Foods: Detailed List of Foods That Promote Gut Healing

A healthy gut is fundamental to overall well-being, as it impacts digestion, immunity, mental health, and even hormone balance. If you're dealing with issues like **leaky gut syndrome, chronic inflammation**, or **gut dysbiosis**, focusing on foods that actively promote gut healing is essential. Certain nutrient-rich, anti-inflammatory foods can help repair the **intestinal lining**, restore a balanced microbiome, and reduce systemic inflammation.

Here's a detailed list of the top **gut-healing foods**—what they are, why they're beneficial, and how to incorporate them into your diet.

1. Bone Broth

Bone broth is one of the most powerful foods for gut healing. Made by simmering bones (such as chicken, beef, or fish) with water, vegetables, and apple cider vinegar, it is rich in nutrients that support the repair of the gut lining.

Benefits:
- **Collagen and Gelatin**: These proteins strengthen the gut lining by promoting the growth of intestinal cells.
- **Amino Acids**: High levels of **L-glutamine, glycine**, and **proline** help repair damaged intestinal tissues and reduce inflammation.
- **Minerals**: Packed with calcium, magnesium, and potassium for overall health.

How to Use:
- Sip warm bone broth as a soothing drink.
- Use it as a base for soups, stews, or sauces.

2. Fermented Foods

Fermented foods are rich in **probiotics**, the beneficial bacteria that support a healthy gut microbiome. These foods help repopulate the gut with good bacteria, crowding out harmful microbes and improving digestion.

Examples:
- **Yogurt** (unsweetened, full-fat, or Greek-style)
- **Kefir**
- **Sauerkraut**
- **Kimchi**
- **Miso**
- **Tempeh**
- **Pickles** (fermented, not vinegar-based)

Benefits:
- **Restores Microbial Balance**: Introduces beneficial bacteria that promote gut health and reduce dysbiosis.
- **Supports Immune Function**: A healthy microbiome improves immune system regulation.
- **Enhances Nutrient Absorption**: Helps the body break down food more effectively, increasing nutrient availability.

How to Use:
- Add a serving of yogurt or kefir to your breakfast.
- Include sauerkraut or kimchi as a side dish with meals.
- Use miso as a base for soups or marinades.

3. Healthy Fats

Anti-inflammatory fats are essential for gut healing. They help reduce inflammation in the gut lining, support cell membranes, and provide energy for healing.

Examples:
- **Omega-3-rich fats**: Fatty fish (salmon, sardines, mackerel), flaxseeds, chia seeds, walnuts
- **Monounsaturated fats**: Avocados, olive oil, almonds
- **Medium-chain triglycerides (MCTs)**: Coconut oil, MCT oil

Benefits:
- **Reduce Inflammation**: Omega-3 fatty acids and MCTs combat chronic inflammation in the gut.
- **Promote Gut Barrier Repair**: Healthy fats nourish the cells of

the gut lining, aiding repair.
- **Support Hormone Balance**: Essential for regulating hormones that affect digestion and immune responses.

How to Use:
- Drizzle olive oil over salads and roasted vegetables.
- Add chia seeds or flaxseeds to smoothies or oatmeal.
- Use coconut oil for cooking or baking.

4. Fiber-Rich Foods

Fiber acts as a **prebiotic**, feeding the beneficial bacteria in the gut and promoting a healthy microbiome. Soluble fiber, in particular, soothes the gut and supports the production of **short-chain fatty acids (SCFAs)**, which help maintain the integrity of the gut lining.

Examples:
- **Fruits**: Berries, bananas (ripe), apples, pears
- **Vegetables**: Asparagus, artichokes, carrots, zucchini
- **Whole Grains**: Oats, quinoa, millet
- **Legumes**: Lentils, chickpeas, black beans

Benefits:
- **Nourish Good Bacteria**: Prebiotic fibers feed beneficial microbes.
- **Enhance Regularity**: Promotes healthy bowel movements, reducing bloating and discomfort.
- **Support SCFA Production**: SCFAs reduce inflammation and strengthen the gut lining.

How to Use:
- Include a variety of fruits and vegetables in every meal.
- Add oats to smoothies or yogurt for a fiber boost.
- Pair legumes with lean proteins for a hearty, gut-healthy meal.

5. Anti-Inflammatory Vegetables

Vegetables rich in **antioxidants** and **phytonutrients** help reduce gut inflammation and provide nutrients that support gut healing.

Examples:
- Leafy greens: Spinach, kale, Swiss chard
- Cruciferous vegetables: Broccoli, cauliflower, Brussels sprouts
- Brightly colored vegetables: Sweet potatoes, bell peppers, carrots,

beets

Benefits:
- **Reduce Oxidative Stress**: Antioxidants in these vegetables combat inflammation in the gut lining.
- **Provide Vitamins and Minerals**: Essential nutrients like vitamin A, C, and magnesium support overall gut health.
- **Boost Fiber Intake**: Adds prebiotic fibers to your diet.

How to Use:
- Steam or sauté vegetables to make them easier to digest.
- Add greens like spinach to smoothies or stir-fries.
- Roast sweet potatoes or carrots as a side dish.

6. Gut-Healing Proteins

Protein is essential for repairing and rebuilding the gut lining. High-quality protein sources provide **amino acids** like **L-glutamine** that directly support intestinal health.

Examples:
- Pasture-raised poultry
- Grass-fed beef
- Wild-caught fish
- Eggs
- Plant-based proteins: Lentils, tofu, tempeh

Benefits:
- **Repair Intestinal Tissue**: Amino acids like glutamine and glycine rebuild the gut lining.
- **Reduce Inflammation**: High-quality protein helps modulate the immune system.
- **Support Digestive Enzyme Production**: Proteins are needed to create enzymes for efficient digestion.

How to Use:
- Include a lean protein source in every meal.
- Use wild-caught fish or poultry as a main dish.
- Add eggs or tempeh to salads for a protein boost.

7. Healing Spices and Herbs

Certain herbs and spices have natural **anti-inflammatory** and **antimicrobial** properties that support gut healing.

Examples:
- Turmeric (with black pepper to enhance absorption)
- Ginger
- Garlic (cooked to reduce harshness)
- Cinnamon
- Oregano

Benefits:
- **Reduce Gut Inflammation**: Compounds like curcumin (in turmeric) and gingerol (in ginger) soothe the gut lining.
- **Support Digestion**: Spices like cinnamon and garlic stimulate digestive enzymes.
- **Combat Harmful Bacteria**: Antimicrobial properties help restore microbial balance.

How to Use:
- Add turmeric and ginger to teas or smoothies.
- Use garlic and oregano to flavor dishes like soups and stews.
- Sprinkle cinnamon on oatmeal or roasted vegetables.

8. Hydrating Beverages

Proper hydration is essential for digestion and gut healing. Certain beverages also have added benefits for soothing the gut lining and reducing inflammation.

Examples:
- Herbal teas: Peppermint, chamomile, ginger, licorice root
- Aloe vera juice (unsweetened)
- Coconut water (unsweetened)

Benefits:
- **Soothe the Gut Lining**: Herbal teas reduce inflammation and calm the digestive tract.
- **Promote Regularity**: Aloe vera juice aids in digestion and reduces constipation.
- **Hydrate**: Proper hydration supports cellular repair and nutrient transport.

How to Use:
- Sip on herbal teas throughout the day.
- Add a splash of aloe vera juice to water or smoothies.

The Leaky Gut Diet: A Comprehensive Guide to an Anti-Inflammatory Diet, Foods to Avoid, and Recipes

The **leaky gut diet** is designed to reduce inflammation, repair the gut lining, and restore balance to the gut microbiome. By eliminating foods that irritate the intestinal lining and prioritizing those that promote healing, this dietary approach can help address the root causes of leaky gut syndrome. The focus is on an **anti-inflammatory diet** rich in nutrient-dense, whole foods while avoiding common irritants such as **gluten, dairy, processed sugars**, and **highly processed foods**.

This guide provides a detailed overview of the leaky gut diet, including foods to avoid, foods to include, and some simple recipes to get started.

1. Principles of the Leaky Gut Diet

The leaky gut diet follows three core principles to promote healing:

1. **Eliminate Inflammatory Foods**:
    - Remove foods that irritate the gut lining, promote inflammation, or disrupt the gut microbiome.
2. **Incorporate Healing Foods**:
    - Prioritize nutrient-dense foods that repair the gut lining, reduce inflammation, and support beneficial gut bacteria.
3. **Focus on Digestive Support**:
    - Choose foods that are easy to digest and promote regular bowel movements while avoiding foods that cause bloating, gas, or discomfort.

2. Foods to Avoid on the Leaky Gut Diet

Certain foods are known to irritate the gut lining, increase inflammation, and exacerbate symptoms of leaky gut syndrome. Eliminating these foods is critical for gut healing.

a. Gluten
- Found in wheat, barley, rye, and many processed foods, **gluten** increases intestinal permeability in sensitive individuals by stimulating the release of **zonulin**, a protein that loosens the tight junctions in the gut lining.

b. Dairy
- Many people with leaky gut are sensitive to **lactose** or **casein**, the sugar and protein in dairy, respectively. These can trigger

inflammation, bloating, and digestive discomfort.

c. Processed Sugars
- Refined sugars feed harmful gut bacteria and yeast, contributing to **dysbiosis** (microbial imbalance) and inflammation.

d. Artificial Additives
- Additives such as **preservatives, emulsifiers,** and **artificial sweeteners** (e.g., aspartame, sucralose) disrupt the gut microbiome and irritate the gut lining.

e. Processed and Fried Foods
- High in unhealthy fats and trans fats, processed and fried foods contribute to systemic inflammation and oxidative stress.

f. Alcohol
- Alcohol damages the gut lining, disrupts microbial balance, and increases intestinal permeability.

g. Soy and Corn
- These common allergens, particularly when genetically modified, may cause inflammation and contribute to gut irritation.

h. Nightshades (for some individuals)
- Vegetables like tomatoes, potatoes, eggplants, and peppers contain **alkaloids** that may trigger inflammation in sensitive individuals.

3. Foods to Include on the Leaky Gut Diet

The leaky gut diet emphasizes foods that are anti-inflammatory, nutrient-dense, and rich in compounds that repair the gut lining and support microbiome health.

a. Healing Proteins
- **Examples**: Pasture-raised poultry, grass-fed beef, wild-caught fish, eggs, lentils, and tempeh.
- **Benefits**: Provide amino acids like **L-glutamine** and **glycine** to repair the intestinal lining.

b. Bone Broth
- **Benefits**: Contains collagen, gelatin, and amino acids that rebuild the gut barrier and reduce inflammation.

c. Fermented Foods
- **Examples**: Yogurt (dairy-free or full-fat unsweetened), kefir,

sauerkraut, kimchi, miso, and tempeh.
- **Benefits**: Rich in probiotics that restore microbial balance and reduce gut inflammation.

d. High-Fiber Foods
- **Examples**: Berries, leafy greens, asparagus, artichokes, and flaxseeds.
- **Benefits**: Act as prebiotics, feeding beneficial gut bacteria and supporting digestion.

e. Anti-Inflammatory Fats
- **Examples**: Avocados, olive oil, coconut oil, and omega-3-rich fatty fish (salmon, mackerel).
- **Benefits**: Reduce systemic inflammation and support cell repair.

f. Vegetables
- **Examples**: Sweet potatoes, zucchini, carrots, beets, spinach, and kale.
- **Benefits**: Packed with antioxidants, vitamins, and minerals that reduce inflammation and support gut health.

g. Herbs and Spices
- **Examples**: Turmeric, ginger, garlic, oregano, and cinnamon.
- **Benefits**: Contain anti-inflammatory and antimicrobial properties.

h. Hydrating Beverages
- **Examples**: Herbal teas (chamomile, peppermint, ginger), coconut water, and aloe vera juice.
- **Benefits**: Soothe the gut lining and support hydration for cellular repair.

4. Sample Recipes for the Leaky Gut Diet

Here are some simple and delicious recipes that align with the principles of the leaky gut diet.

a. Healing Bone Broth Soup
Ingredients:
- 2 cups bone broth
- 1 cup shredded chicken
- 1 cup chopped spinach
- 1 medium zucchini, spiralized or chopped

- 1 clove garlic, minced
- 1 tsp turmeric
- 1 tsp olive oil
- Salt and pepper to taste

Instructions:
1. Heat olive oil in a pot over medium heat. Sauté garlic until fragrant.
2. Add bone broth and bring to a simmer.
3. Stir in shredded chicken, spinach, zucchini, and turmeric.
4. Simmer for 5-7 minutes until vegetables are tender.
5. Season with salt and pepper before serving.

b. Gut-Healing Smoothie
Ingredients:
- 1 cup unsweetened almond milk
- ½ cup frozen blueberries
- 1 ripe banana
- 1 tbsp chia seeds
- 1 tbsp coconut oil
- ½ tsp cinnamon

Instructions:
1. Combine all ingredients in a blender.
2. Blend until smooth.
3. Serve immediately for a nourishing, gut-friendly breakfast or snack.

c. Roasted Sweet Potato and Avocado Salad
Ingredients:
- 2 medium sweet potatoes, diced
- 1 tbsp coconut oil
- 2 cups mixed greens
- 1 avocado, sliced
- 2 tbsp olive oil
- 1 tsp lemon juice
- Salt and pepper to taste

Instructions:
1. Preheat the oven to 400°F (200°C). Toss sweet potatoes with

coconut oil and roast for 20-25 minutes until tender.
2. In a bowl, combine mixed greens, roasted sweet potatoes, and avocado slices.
3. Drizzle with olive oil and lemon juice. Season with salt and pepper.

d. Turmeric Ginger Tea
Ingredients:
- 1 cup hot water
- 1 tsp turmeric powder
- 1 tsp grated ginger
- ½ tsp cinnamon
- 1 tsp raw honey (optional)

Instructions:
1. Add turmeric, ginger, and cinnamon to hot water. Stir well.
2. Let steep for 5 minutes.
3. Sweeten with raw honey if desired. Sip and enjoy.

5. Practical Tips for Success
1. **Meal Prep**: Plan meals ahead to avoid reaching for processed or inflammatory foods.
2. **Elimination Diet**: Identify and remove personal trigger foods, such as gluten or dairy, by reintroducing them after a period of elimination.
3. **Listen to Your Body**: Pay attention to how your body responds to specific foods and adjust your diet accordingly.
4. **Stay Hydrated**: Drink plenty of water and herbal teas to support digestion and nutrient absorption.

Supplements for Gut Health: Top Supplements to Support Healing and Digestion

A balanced diet rich in gut-healing foods is essential for repairing the gut lining and restoring a healthy microbiome. However, supplements can play a crucial role in accelerating gut healing, reducing inflammation, and improving digestion. When chosen carefully, supplements like **L-glutamine, probiotics**, and **digestive enzymes** can enhance your body's ability to repair and maintain optimal gut health.

In this section, we'll explore the **top supplements for gut health**, how they work, their benefits, and tips for choosing and incorporating them into your routine.

1. L-Glutamine

L-glutamine is an amino acid that serves as a primary fuel source for the cells lining the gut (enterocytes). It is one of the most effective supplements for repairing the **intestinal barrier** and reducing gut inflammation.

How It Works:
- **Repairs the Gut Lining**: L-glutamine strengthens the tight junctions between intestinal cells, helping to seal the gut lining and reduce intestinal permeability.
- **Reduces Inflammation**: It calms gut inflammation, which is critical for healing conditions like **leaky gut syndrome**.
- **Supports Immune Function**: As a key fuel for immune cells in the gut, it helps maintain a healthy balance between tolerance and immune defense.

Benefits:
- Repairs the gut lining in cases of leaky gut.
- Reduces symptoms of bloating, gas, and digestive discomfort.
- Enhances recovery from chronic stress or illnesses that weaken gut health.

How to Use:
- Dosage: **5-10 grams per day**, divided into 2-3 doses. Start with lower doses and increase as tolerated.
- Form: Available as a powder or capsule. Mix the powder in water or smoothies for easy consumption.
- Timing: Take on an empty stomach for best absorption.

2. Probiotics

Probiotics are live microorganisms (beneficial bacteria) that help restore balance to the gut microbiome, improving digestion and reducing inflammation. They are particularly effective for addressing **dysbiosis** (an imbalance of gut bacteria).

How They Work:
- **Restore Microbial Balance**: Probiotics increase the population of good bacteria, crowding out harmful microbes that disrupt gut

health.
- **Support the Immune System**: They help regulate immune responses, reducing excessive inflammation.
- **Aid Digestion**: Probiotics break down complex carbohydrates and fibers that would otherwise cause bloating and gas.

Benefits:
- Improve digestion and reduce symptoms of IBS, like bloating and diarrhea.
- Enhance immune function by strengthening the gut barrier.
- Promote mental well-being by supporting the gut-brain axis.

Best Strains for Gut Health:
- **Lactobacillus acidophilus**: Supports digestion and reduces inflammation.
- **Bifidobacterium bifidum**: Improves gut barrier integrity and enhances immune function.
- **Saccharomyces boulardii**: Effective for managing diarrhea and restoring microbiome balance after antibiotic use.

How to Use:
- Dosage: **10-20 billion CFUs (colony-forming units)** per day for maintenance; higher doses may be needed for specific conditions.
- Form: Capsules, powders, or fermented food supplements.
- Timing: Take with meals to protect the probiotics from stomach acid.

3. Digestive Enzymes

Digestive enzymes are natural proteins that help break down food into smaller, absorbable nutrients. For individuals with compromised digestion, supplementing with digestive enzymes can reduce stress on the gut and improve nutrient absorption.

How They Work:
- **Enhance Digestion**: Digestive enzymes break down proteins, fats, carbohydrates, and fibers, preventing undigested food particles from irritating the gut lining.
- **Reduce Bloating**: By aiding digestion, they minimize gas and bloating caused by poor food breakdown.

- **Support Nutrient Absorption**: Proper digestion ensures that your body absorbs the vitamins and minerals needed for gut repair.

Benefits:
- Alleviate symptoms of indigestion, gas, and bloating.
- Reduce food sensitivities by assisting in breaking down common irritants like lactose or gluten.
- Improve energy levels by enhancing nutrient absorption.

Key Enzymes:
- **Protease**: Breaks down proteins into amino acids.
- **Amylase**: Breaks down carbohydrates into sugars.
- **Lipase**: Breaks down fats into fatty acids.
- **Lactase**: Helps digest lactose, the sugar in dairy.

How to Use:
- Dosage: Follow the manufacturer's instructions (typically 1-2 capsules per meal).
- Timing: Take immediately before or during meals for maximum effectiveness.
- Form: Available as capsules or powders.

4. Collagen Peptides

Collagen peptides are broken-down forms of collagen protein that are easily absorbed by the body. They are rich in amino acids like **glycine** and **proline**, which are essential for gut repair.

How It Works:
- **Rebuilds Gut Lining**: Collagen strengthens the gut barrier by supporting the structural integrity of the intestinal wall.
- **Reduces Inflammation**: Glycine in collagen has anti-inflammatory properties that calm the gut lining.
- **Promotes Tissue Repair**: Accelerates the healing of damaged tissues in the gut.

Benefits:
- Enhances gut barrier function to reduce intestinal permeability.
- Improves skin, hair, and joint health as an added benefit.
- Soothes inflammation in the digestive tract.

How to Use:

- Dosage: **10-20 grams per day**.
- Form: Powder that dissolves easily in hot or cold liquids.
- Timing: Add to coffee, tea, smoothies, or soups.

5. Zinc Carnosine

Zinc carnosine is a unique combination of zinc and carnosine that specifically supports gut health and healing.

How It Works:

- **Protects the Gut Lining**: It forms a protective barrier on the gut lining, shielding it from damage.
- **Supports Cellular Repair**: Zinc promotes the growth and repair of gut cells.
- **Reduces Inflammation**: It modulates inflammatory responses in the gut.

Benefits:

- Helps heal ulcers and gut lining damage.
- Reduces symptoms of heartburn and gastritis.
- Improves gut barrier integrity.

How to Use:

- Dosage: **75-150 mg per day**, divided into two doses.
- Timing: Take with meals.
- Form: Capsules or tablets.

6. Slippery Elm and Marshmallow Root

These natural supplements are mucilaginous herbs that coat the gut lining, reducing irritation and promoting healing.

How They Work:

- **Soothe and Protect**: Form a protective layer over the gut lining, reducing inflammation and preventing damage from stomach acid or irritants.
- **Stimulate Mucus Production**: Enhance mucus secretion, which helps protect and heal the intestinal lining.

Benefits:

- Relieve symptoms of acid reflux, heartburn, and gastritis.
- Calm irritated gut tissue.
- Support overall digestive health.

How to Use:

- Dosage: **1-2 teaspoons of powder** mixed with water or tea, 1-3 times daily.
- Timing: Take before meals for maximum soothing effect.
- Form: Available as powders, capsules, or teas.

7. Aloe Vera

Aloe vera is a natural anti-inflammatory and soothing agent that supports digestion and gut healing.

How It Works:
- **Calms Inflammation**: Reduces irritation in the gut lining.
- **Supports Digestion**: Enhances nutrient absorption and bowel regularity.
- **Promotes Healing**: Contains compounds that accelerate tissue repair.

Benefits:
- Eases symptoms of IBS, acid reflux, and leaky gut.
- Improves hydration in the digestive tract.
- Promotes regular bowel movements.

How to Use:
- Dosage: **1-2 tablespoons of aloe vera juice**, up to twice daily.
- Timing: Take before meals.
- Form: Choose pure, unsweetened aloe vera juice.

8. Omega-3 Fatty Acids

Omega-3 fatty acids, found in fish oil and flaxseed oil, are potent anti-inflammatory agents that support gut healing.

How They Work:
- **Reduce Inflammation**: Lower the production of inflammatory cytokines in the gut.
- **Support Cell Repair**: Strengthen intestinal cells and improve barrier function.

Benefits:
- Improve symptoms of IBS, colitis, and other inflammatory gut conditions.
- Support the growth of beneficial bacteria in the gut.

How to Use:
- Dosage: **1-2 grams per day**.

- Form: Fish oil capsules or liquid, or flaxseed oil.
- Timing: Take with meals.

Tips for Choosing and Using Gut Health Supplements
1. **Choose High-Quality Products:**
    - Look for third-party testing or certification to ensure purity and potency.
    - Avoid supplements with unnecessary fillers or additives.
2. **Start Slowly:**
    - Introduce one supplement at a time to monitor how your body reacts.
    - Gradually increase the dosage as needed.
3. **Consult a Healthcare Professional:**
    - If you have underlying health conditions or are on medication, consult your doctor or a nutritionist before starting new supplements.
4. **Combine with a Gut-Healing Diet:**
    - Supplements work best when paired with an anti-inflammatory diet rich in whole, nutrient-dense foods.

Chapter 6: A 30-Day Leaky Gut Healing Plan for Women

Healing leaky gut requires a structured and consistent approach that integrates **dietary changes**, **lifestyle modifications**, and **targeted supplementation**. A 30-day plan can help you kickstart the healing process, providing your gut the time and tools it needs to repair, reduce inflammation, and restore balance to your microbiome. This plan is tailored specifically for women, taking into account common hormonal imbalances and unique health challenges.

Overview of the 30-Day Plan
Goals:
1. Reduce inflammation and soothe the gut lining.
2. Eliminate foods that irritate the gut or disrupt hormonal balance.
3. Incorporate nutrient-dense, gut-healing foods.
4. Support gut repair with supplements and stress management.

Key Components:
- **Phase 1 (Days 1–10)**: Elimination and Detoxification
- **Phase 2 (Days 11–20)**: Repair and Rebuild
- **Phase 3 (Days 21–30)**: Strengthen and Sustain

Phase 1: Elimination and Detoxification (Days 1–10)
This phase focuses on removing gut irritants and inflammatory

triggers while introducing gentle detoxification practices to support gut repair.

What to Eliminate:
- **Gluten**: Found in wheat, barley, and rye.
- **Dairy**: Including milk, cheese, and yogurt (opt for non-dairy alternatives).
- **Processed Sugars**: Refined sugars and artificial sweeteners.
- **Alcohol**: All forms of alcoholic beverages.
- **Processed Foods**: Packaged snacks, fast foods, and preservatives.
- **Caffeine**: Limit coffee and caffeinated beverages.

Foods to Emphasize:
- **Bone Broth**: Rich in collagen and amino acids for gut repair.
- **Steamed Vegetables**: Easy-to-digest options like zucchini, carrots, and spinach.
- **Lean Proteins**: Organic chicken, turkey, and wild-caught fish.
- **Fermented Foods**: Small amounts of sauerkraut or kimchi to introduce probiotics.
- **Healthy Fats**: Avocados, olive oil, and coconut oil.

Detoxification Practices:
- **Hydration**: Drink at least 8–10 glasses of water daily, infused with lemon for added detox support.
- **Herbal Teas**: Chamomile, peppermint, or ginger tea to soothe the digestive tract.
- **Light Exercise**: Yoga or gentle walking to promote lymphatic flow.

Sample Day:
- **Breakfast**: Gut-Healing Smoothie (almond milk, frozen berries, chia seeds, and collagen peptides).
- **Lunch**: Grilled salmon with steamed broccoli and sweet potato.
- **Snack**: Sliced cucumber with guacamole.
- **Dinner**: Chicken bone broth soup with zucchini noodles and shredded carrots.
- **Supplement**: L-glutamine (5g), probiotics (10 billion CFUs).

Phase 2: Repair and Rebuild (Days 11–20)

This phase focuses on actively repairing the gut lining and introducing more diverse foods to rebuild microbial balance.

Focus Areas:
- **Increased Fiber:** Add prebiotic foods like asparagus, bananas, and garlic to feed beneficial gut bacteria.
- **Anti-Inflammatory Foods:** Incorporate turmeric, ginger, and leafy greens.
- **Probiotic Diversity:** Increase the variety of fermented foods like kefir, miso, and coconut yogurt.

Foods to Introduce:
- **Root Vegetables:** Sweet potatoes, beets, and parsnips for nutrient support.
- **Nuts and Seeds:** Chia seeds, flaxseeds, and almonds in moderation.
- **Additional Proteins:** Eggs and legumes (if tolerated).

Lifestyle Tips:
- **Sleep Hygiene:** Aim for 7–9 hours of quality sleep per night.
- **Mindfulness:** Practice meditation or deep breathing to reduce cortisol levels.

Sample Day:
- **Breakfast:** Scrambled eggs with sautéed spinach and avocado slices.
- **Lunch:** Mixed greens with grilled chicken, roasted beets, and olive oil dressing.
- **Snack:** Coconut yogurt with a sprinkle of flaxseeds.
- **Dinner:** Baked cod with asparagus and mashed sweet potatoes.
- **Supplement:** Digestive enzymes with meals, collagen peptides (10g).

Phase 3: Strengthen and Sustain (Days 21–30)

The final phase is about maintaining progress, increasing food variety, and establishing habits for long-term gut health.

Focus Areas:
- **Expand Diet:** Slowly reintroduce foods like legumes, nightshades, or gluten-free grains (quinoa, millet) while monitoring symptoms.

- **Optimize Microbiome**: Continue with prebiotic and probiotic-rich foods.
- **Long-Term Strategies**: Develop sustainable routines for meal prep, stress management, and sleep.

Foods to Introduce:
- **Gluten-Free Grains**: Quinoa, millet, or buckwheat.
- **Fruits**: Apples, pears, and citrus fruits in moderation.
- **Lean Meats**: Grass-fed beef and organic turkey.

Lifestyle Tips:
- **Regular Exercise**: Incorporate moderate-intensity activities like Pilates or swimming.
- **Track Progress**: Keep a journal of symptoms, energy levels, and digestion.

Sample Day:
- **Breakfast**: Quinoa porridge with almond milk, cinnamon, and sliced bananas.
- **Lunch**: Grass-fed beef burger on a bed of greens with roasted vegetables.
- **Snack**: Handful of walnuts and a sliced apple.
- **Dinner**: Herb-roasted chicken with sautéed Brussels sprouts and quinoa.
- **Supplement**: Omega-3 (1–2g), probiotics (20 billion CFUs).

Supplements for Each Phase

Phase 1:
- L-glutamine (5g daily): Repairs the gut lining.
- Probiotics (10 billion CFUs): Replenish beneficial bacteria.

Phase 2:
- Digestive enzymes: Improve nutrient absorption.
- Collagen peptides (10–20g daily): Strengthen the intestinal barrier.

Phase 3:
- Omega-3 fatty acids (1–2g daily): Reduce inflammation.
- Zinc carnosine (75mg daily): Support gut lining repair.

Tracking Your Progress

To measure the effectiveness of the 30-day plan, keep track of:

- **Digestive Symptoms**: Bloating, gas, constipation, or diarrhea.
- **Energy Levels**: Fatigue and mental clarity.
- **Skin and Inflammation**: Reductions in acne, eczema, or joint pain.
- **Hormonal Health**: Improvements in PMS symptoms or menstrual regularity.

Step-by-Step Protocol: A 30-Day Healing Program for Gut Health

This **30-day healing program** offers a comprehensive, daily step-by-step guide to heal **leaky gut syndrome** and restore gut health. The protocol combines **dietary changes, exercise routines**, and **mindfulness practices** for holistic healing. It is broken into three phases: **Detox and Elimination, Repair and Rebuild**, and **Strengthen and Maintain**. Each phase is designed to target specific aspects of gut healing, ensuring sustainable progress.

Phase 1: Detox and Elimination (Days 1–10)

This phase focuses on removing gut irritants, reducing inflammation, and preparing the body for repair. You'll follow a clean, anti-inflammatory diet, start gentle movement routines, and introduce stress management practices.

Daily Schedule
Morning:
1. **Hydrate**: Drink a glass of warm water with lemon to stimulate digestion and detoxify.
2. **Breakfast**: A gut-healing smoothie:
    - Unsweetened almond milk
    - 1 scoop of collagen peptides
    - ½ cup frozen berries
    - 1 tbsp chia seeds
    - 1 tsp coconut oil
3. **Supplement**: Take **L-glutamine (5g)** to repair the gut lining.

Mid-Morning:
- Optional snack: Cucumber slices with guacamole.
- Gentle **stretching or yoga**: 10–15 minutes of poses like Cat-Cow and Child's Pose to reduce stress and improve circulation.

Lunch:
- Grilled chicken or wild-caught salmon with steamed broccoli and roasted sweet potato.
- Drizzle with olive oil or coconut oil for healthy fats.
- Optional herbal tea (peppermint or chamomile) to aid digestion.

Afternoon:
- **Mindfulness Practice**: Spend 5–10 minutes meditating or practicing deep breathing.
- Snack: Handful of almonds or a small serving of sauerkraut for probiotics.

Dinner:
- Bone broth soup with zucchini noodles, shredded carrots, and fresh parsley.
- Sprinkle with turmeric and ginger for anti-inflammatory benefits.

Evening:
1. **Relaxation Ritual**: Take a warm Epsom salt bath to promote detoxification and stress relief.
2. **Supplement**: Take **probiotics (10 billion CFUs)** and a cup of ginger tea to soothe the digestive system.

Phase 2: Repair and Rebuild (Days 11–20)

This phase emphasizes foods and practices that actively repair the gut lining and support microbial balance. You'll build on the foundation from Phase 1 by incorporating more fiber-rich and probiotic foods.

Daily Schedule

Morning:
1. **Hydrate**: Start with water infused with cucumber and mint to refresh the system.
2. **Breakfast**: Scrambled eggs with sautéed spinach and avocado slices.
3. **Supplement**: Continue **L-glutamine (5g)** and add **digestive enzymes** with meals to improve nutrient absorption.

Mid-Morning:
- Optional snack: Coconut yogurt with a sprinkle of flaxseeds.
- **Gentle Exercise**: A brisk 15–20 minute walk or light yoga.

Lunch:

- Grilled turkey burger on a bed of mixed greens, roasted beets, and olive oil vinaigrette.
- Side of fermented vegetables like kimchi or sauerkraut for probiotics.

Afternoon:
- **Mindfulness Practice**: Journaling for 10 minutes to reflect on progress and emotional well-being.
- Snack: A sliced apple with almond butter or a small handful of walnuts.

Dinner:
- Herb-roasted chicken with mashed cauliflower and steamed asparagus.
- Sip on bone broth for an extra dose of collagen.

Evening:
1. **Relaxation Ritual**: Read or meditate with calming music for 15–20 minutes.
2. **Supplement**: Continue **probiotics** and add **collagen peptides (10g)** to a warm herbal tea.

Phase 3: Strengthen and Maintain (Days 21–30)

This phase focuses on long-term maintenance, introducing more food variety, and solidifying healthy habits for gut health.

Daily Schedule

Morning:
1. **Hydrate**: Start the day with water and a pinch of Himalayan salt for hydration.
2. **Breakfast**: Quinoa porridge with almond milk, cinnamon, and sliced bananas.
3. **Supplement**: Take **L-glutamine (5g)** and **omega-3 fatty acids (1–2g)** for anti-inflammatory support.

Mid-Morning:
- Optional snack: Hard-boiled egg with a sprinkle of sea salt.
- **Moderate Exercise**: 20–30 minutes of Pilates, swimming, or a nature walk.

Lunch:
- Grass-fed beef burger with roasted Brussels sprouts and mashed

sweet potatoes.
- Add sauerkraut or pickled carrots for gut-friendly probiotics.

Afternoon:
- **Mindfulness Practice**: Try a 5-minute gratitude meditation to reduce cortisol and improve overall well-being.
- Snack: Handful of pumpkin seeds or a small serving of coconut yogurt.

Dinner:
- Baked salmon with a side of quinoa and roasted zucchini.
- Garnish with fresh herbs like parsley and dill for added antioxidants.

Evening:
1. **Wind-Down Routine**: Practice progressive muscle relaxation for stress relief.
2. **Supplement**: Probiotics and magnesium citrate (200-400 mg) to promote relaxation and bowel regularity.

Additional Protocols

Weekly Detox Practice
- Incorporate a half-day fast (e.g., consuming only bone broth, herbal teas, and water) once a week to give the gut a break and support detoxification.

Reintroducing Foods (Optional in Phase 3)
- Slowly reintroduce potentially triggering foods like legumes, gluten-free grains, or nightshades.
- Add one food every 3–5 days while monitoring symptoms.

Key Supplements for Each Phase

Phase	Supplement	Purpose
Phase 1	L-glutamine (5g/day)	Repairs gut lining and reduces inflammation.
	Probiotics (10 billion CFUs)	Replenishes beneficial gut bacteria.

Phase	Supplement	Purpose
Phase 2	Digestive enzymes	Improves digestion and nutrient absorption.
	Collagen peptides (10g/day)	Supports gut lining integrity and tissue repair.
Phase 3	Omega-3 fatty acids (1-2g)	Reduces inflammation and supports microbial balance.
	Magnesium citrate	Relieves constipation and promotes relaxation.

Daily Meal Plans: Easy-to-Follow Recipes for Gut Healing and Reducing Inflammation

When healing leaky gut, having a **structured meal plan** can make all the difference. A daily plan with nutrient-dense, anti-inflammatory recipes ensures your body gets the nutrients it needs to repair the gut lining, rebalance the microbiome, and reduce inflammation. Below, you'll find easy-to-follow meal plans with recipes tailored to promote gut healing and improve digestion.

Day 1: Simple and Nourishing
Breakfast: Gut-Healing Smoothie
Ingredients:
- 1 cup unsweetened almond milk
- ½ cup frozen blueberries
- 1 ripe banana
- 1 scoop collagen peptides
- 1 tbsp chia seeds
- 1 tsp coconut oil

Instructions:
1. Combine all ingredients in a blender.
2. Blend until smooth.
3. Serve immediately.

Benefits: This smoothie is packed with gut-healing collagen, fiber from chia seeds, and anti-inflammatory antioxidants from blueberries.

Lunch: Herb-Roasted Salmon with Steamed Broccoli
Ingredients:
- 1 salmon fillet (wild-caught)
- 1 tsp olive oil
- 1 tsp dried dill or parsley
- 1 cup broccoli florets
- 1 tsp lemon juice
- Salt and pepper to taste

Instructions:
1. Preheat oven to 375°F (190°C).
2. Rub the salmon with olive oil, dill, salt, and pepper.
3. Bake for 15–20 minutes until fully cooked.
4. Steam broccoli until tender and drizzle with lemon juice.
5. Serve with the salmon.

Benefits: Salmon provides omega-3 fatty acids to reduce inflammation, while broccoli contains prebiotic fiber to nourish gut bacteria.

Snack: Coconut Yogurt with Flaxseeds
Ingredients:
- ½ cup unsweetened coconut yogurt
- 1 tbsp ground flaxseeds
- 1 tsp raw honey (optional)

Instructions:
1. Mix flaxseeds into the coconut yogurt.
2. Drizzle with raw honey if desired.

Benefits: Probiotics in yogurt help restore microbial balance, and flaxseeds provide omega-3s and prebiotic fiber.

Dinner: Bone Broth Chicken Soup with Vegetables
Ingredients:
- 2 cups chicken bone broth
- 1 cup shredded chicken (cooked)
- 1 cup zucchini noodles
- ½ cup diced carrots
- 1 clove garlic, minced

- 1 tsp turmeric
- Salt and pepper to taste

Instructions:
1. Heat bone broth in a pot over medium heat.
2. Add carrots, garlic, and turmeric. Simmer for 10 minutes.
3. Stir in chicken and zucchini noodles. Cook for another 5 minutes.
4. Season with salt and pepper. Serve warm.

Benefits: Bone broth contains collagen and amino acids like L-glutamine to repair the gut lining, while turmeric adds anti-inflammatory properties.

Day 2: Anti-Inflammatory Favorites
Breakfast: Sweet Potato Breakfast Bowl
Ingredients:
- 1 medium sweet potato (baked or steamed)
- 1 tbsp almond butter
- 1 tsp cinnamon
- 1 tbsp crushed walnuts
- 1 tsp raw honey (optional)

Instructions:
1. Mash the sweet potato and place in a bowl.
2. Drizzle with almond butter and sprinkle with cinnamon and walnuts.
3. Add raw honey if desired.

Benefits: Sweet potatoes are easy to digest and rich in fiber, while almond butter and walnuts provide healthy fats.

Lunch: Turkey and Avocado Salad
Ingredients:
- 2 cups mixed greens
- 3–4 slices turkey breast (organic, nitrate-free)
- ½ avocado, sliced
- 1 tbsp olive oil
- 1 tsp apple cider vinegar
- Salt and pepper to taste

Instructions:

1. Arrange greens, turkey, and avocado on a plate.
2. Drizzle with olive oil and apple cider vinegar.
3. Season with salt and pepper.

Benefits: This salad is packed with lean protein, healthy fats, and anti-inflammatory greens.

Snack: Carrot Sticks with Tahini Dip

Ingredients:
- 1 cup carrot sticks
- 2 tbsp tahini
- 1 tsp lemon juice
- 1 pinch garlic powder

Instructions:
1. Mix tahini, lemon juice, and garlic powder in a small bowl.
2. Use carrot sticks for dipping.

Benefits: Carrots are prebiotic-rich, while tahini provides gut-supportive magnesium and healthy fats.

Dinner: Zucchini and Cauliflower Stir-Fry with Shrimp

Ingredients:
- 1 cup shrimp (peeled and deveined)
- 1 medium zucchini, sliced
- 1 cup cauliflower rice
- 1 clove garlic, minced
- 1 tbsp coconut oil
- 1 tsp grated ginger
- 1 tsp coconut aminos (optional)

Instructions:
1. Heat coconut oil in a pan over medium heat.
2. Sauté garlic and ginger for 1 minute.
3. Add shrimp and cook until pink.
4. Stir in zucchini and cauliflower rice. Cook until tender.
5. Drizzle with coconut aminos before serving.

Benefits: This stir-fry is anti-inflammatory, low-carb, and packed with fiber and protein.

Day 3: Variety and Flavor

Breakfast: Collagen Matcha Latte and Scrambled Eggs

Ingredients for Latte:
- 1 cup unsweetened almond milk
- 1 tsp matcha powder
- 1 scoop collagen peptides
- 1 tsp raw honey

Instructions:
1. Heat almond milk until warm but not boiling.
2. Whisk in matcha powder, collagen, and honey until frothy.
3. Serve immediately.

Ingredients for Eggs:
- 2 eggs (pasture-raised)
- 1 tsp olive oil
- 1 tbsp chopped parsley

Instructions:
1. Heat olive oil in a pan over medium heat.
2. Scramble eggs until fully cooked. Garnish with parsley.

Benefits: The matcha latte provides antioxidants, while collagen and eggs support gut repair.

Lunch: Mediterranean Bowl

Ingredients:
- 1 cup cooked quinoa
- ½ cup roasted chickpeas
- ½ cup chopped cucumber
- ½ cup cherry tomatoes
- 1 tbsp tahini dressing
- 1 tsp fresh dill or parsley

Instructions:
1. Arrange all ingredients in a bowl.
2. Drizzle with tahini dressing and garnish with herbs.

Benefits: Quinoa and chickpeas provide fiber and plant-based protein, while tahini adds healthy fats.

Snack: Apple Slices with Sunflower Seed Butter

Ingredients:
- 1 apple, sliced
- 2 tbsp sunflower seed butter

Instructions:
1. Dip apple slices into sunflower seed butter.
2. Enjoy as a quick and satisfying snack.

Benefits: This snack is high in fiber, vitamin C, and healthy fats, supporting digestion and gut healing.

Dinner: Herb-Rubbed Chicken with Roasted Vegetables

Ingredients:
- 1 chicken breast
- 1 tsp dried rosemary
- 1 tsp olive oil
- 1 cup roasted vegetables (sweet potatoes, zucchini, and carrots)
- Salt and pepper to taste

Instructions:
1. Preheat oven to 375°F (190°C).
2. Rub chicken breast with olive oil, rosemary, salt, and pepper.
3. Bake for 20–25 minutes until fully cooked.
4. Roast vegetables alongside chicken, tossing with olive oil and seasoning.

Benefits: This balanced meal provides lean protein, anti-inflammatory fats, and gut-friendly fiber.

Tips for Success
1. **Plan Ahead**: Prepare ingredients like bone broth, roasted vegetables, and proteins in advance to save time.
2. **Hydration**: Drink herbal teas like chamomile or peppermint between meals to soothe digestion.
3. **Customize**: Adjust portion sizes and ingredients based on your preferences and tolerance levels.

Mind-Body Practices: Reducing Stress for Optimal Gut Healing

Stress has a profound impact on gut health. Chronic stress disrupts the gut-brain axis, increases intestinal permeability (leaky gut), and alters the gut microbiome, leading to inflammation and digestive issues. Incorporating **mind-body practices** like yoga, meditation, and journaling can significantly reduce stress, support gut healing, and improve overall well-being. These practices address both the physical and emotional aspects of gut health, making them essential components of a holistic healing approach.

1. Yoga: Gentle Movement for Gut Health

Yoga is a powerful practice for promoting relaxation, improving digestion, and enhancing circulation to the abdominal organs. Specific poses and breathing exercises in yoga stimulate the parasympathetic nervous system, also known as the "rest-and-digest" mode, which is crucial for gut repair and overall digestive health.

Benefits of Yoga for Gut Healing

- **Reduces Stress**: Yoga lowers cortisol levels, reducing gut inflammation caused by chronic stress.
- **Improves Digestion**: Gentle twists and stretches stimulate the digestive organs, enhancing peristalsis (the movement of food through the gut).
- **Boosts Circulation**: Increased blood flow to the abdominal region supports nutrient absorption and gut repair.

Key Yoga Poses for Gut Healing

1. **Child's Pose (Balasana)**:
   - Soothes the nervous system and relaxes the abdominal muscles.
   - Helps alleviate bloating and gas.
   - **How to Do It**: Kneel on the mat, sit back on your heels, and stretch your arms forward while resting your forehead on the mat.

2. **Cat-Cow Pose (Marjaryasana-Bitilasana)**:
   - Improves spinal flexibility and massages the digestive organs.
   - Enhances the connection between breath and movement, calming the mind.
   - **How to Do It**: Alternate between arching your back (Cow) and rounding your spine (Cat) on hands and knees.

3. **Supine Twist (Supta Matsyendrasana)**:
   - Stimulates the digestive organs and aids in detoxification.
   - Relieves tension in the lower back and abdomen.
   - **How to Do It**: Lie on your back, bend one knee, and

twist it across your body while keeping your shoulders on the mat.
4. **Seated Forward Fold (Paschimottanasana)**:
    - Promotes relaxation and stretches the digestive tract.
    - **How to Do It**: Sit on the floor with your legs extended, hinge at the hips, and reach for your feet.

Incorporating Yoga into Your Routine
- **Frequency**: Aim for 3–4 sessions per week, lasting 20–30 minutes.
- **When to Practice**: Perform gentle poses in the morning to kickstart digestion or in the evening to unwind.

2. Meditation: Calming the Gut-Brain Axis

Meditation is one of the most effective tools for managing stress and supporting gut health. By calming the mind, meditation activates the parasympathetic nervous system, reduces inflammation, and improves gut motility. It also enhances mindfulness, helping you make healthier choices regarding food and lifestyle.

Benefits of Meditation for Gut Healing
- **Lowers Cortisol**: Chronic stress increases cortisol, which can disrupt the gut lining and microbiome. Meditation helps lower these levels.
- **Improves Mind-Gut Communication**: Strengthens the gut-brain axis, reducing symptoms like bloating and abdominal pain.
- **Promotes Mindful Eating**: Encourages awareness of hunger and fullness cues, reducing overeating and improving digestion.

Simple Meditation Practices
1. **Breath Awareness Meditation**:
    - Focus on the natural rhythm of your breath to anchor your mind and reduce stress.
    - **How to Do It**: Sit comfortably, close your eyes, and take slow, deep breaths. Focus on the sensation of air entering and leaving your nostrils.
2. **Body Scan Meditation**:
    - Helps release tension in the body and promote relaxation.

- **How to Do It**: Lie down, close your eyes, and mentally scan your body from head to toe, noticing areas of tension and consciously relaxing them.

3. **Loving-Kindness Meditation**:
    - Reduces negative emotions and promotes self-compassion, which supports overall well-being.
    - **How to Do It**: Sit quietly and silently repeat phrases like "May I be healthy, may I be happy, may I be free from stress," extending these wishes to others as well.

Incorporating Meditation into Your Routine
- **Frequency**: Start with 5–10 minutes daily and gradually increase to 20–30 minutes.
- **When to Practice**: Meditate in the morning to set a calm tone for the day or before bed to promote restful sleep.

3. Journaling: Reflective Writing for Emotional Well-Being

Journaling is a therapeutic practice that helps process emotions, identify stress triggers, and cultivate gratitude. Since stress and emotional health significantly affect gut health, regular journaling can provide clarity and reduce mental strain.

Benefits of Journaling for Gut Healing
- **Identifies Stressors**: Helps pinpoint specific sources of stress that may be impacting gut health.
- **Encourages Emotional Release**: Provides an outlet for processing emotions, reducing stress-induced gut symptoms.
- **Tracks Progress**: Allows you to monitor dietary changes, symptoms, and emotional patterns to better understand your healing journey.

Types of Journaling
1. **Gratitude Journal**:
    - Focuses on positive aspects of your day to shift your mindset and reduce stress.
    - **Prompt**: Write three things you are grateful for each day.
2. **Food and Mood Journal**:
    - Tracks your meals, symptoms, and emotional states to identify patterns.

- **Prompt**: Record what you ate, how you felt physically (e.g., bloated, energetic), and your emotional state.
3. **Stream-of-Consciousness Writing**:
   - Freely write your thoughts without worrying about structure or grammar to release pent-up stress.
   - **Prompt**: Write for 10 minutes about whatever is on your mind.

Incorporating Journaling into Your Routine
- **Frequency**: Write daily or at least 3–4 times per week.
- **When to Practice**: Journal in the evening to reflect on the day or after meals to track food and symptoms.

4. Combining Practices for Maximum Benefit

To maximize the benefits of mind-body practices for gut healing, combine yoga, meditation, and journaling into your daily routine:

Morning Routine (15–20 minutes)
- Start with **Breath Awareness Meditation** for 5 minutes.
- Perform gentle yoga poses like **Cat-Cow** or **Child's Pose** for 10 minutes.
- Write in your **Gratitude Journal** to set a positive tone for the day.

Afternoon Reset (10–15 minutes)
- Take a break for **Body Scan Meditation** to release tension.
- Do a short yoga sequence, focusing on **twists** to aid digestion.

Evening Wind-Down (20–30 minutes)
- Practice a calming yoga flow with **Seated Forward Fold** and **Supine Twist**.
- Meditate using **Loving-Kindness Meditation** to promote relaxation.
- Write in your **Food and Mood Journal** to reflect on your meals and symptoms.

Tracking Progress: How to Monitor Symptoms, Mood, and Energy Levels Throughout the Gut Healing Program

Tracking your progress during a gut healing program is crucial for understanding how your body responds to dietary changes, supplements, and lifestyle practices. By monitoring symptoms, mood, and energy levels, you can identify patterns, measure improvements, and make informed adjustments to your plan. A well-organized tracking system not only keeps you motivated but also provides valuable insights into your healing journey.

This guide will show you how to track key aspects of your health effectively, with specific tools, methods, and tips.

Why Tracking Progress Matters

1. **Identify Triggers**:
   - Tracking helps pinpoint foods, activities, or habits that worsen symptoms, enabling you to eliminate or modify them.
2. **Measure Improvements**:
   - Monitoring changes over time allows you to see tangible results, such as reduced bloating, improved mood, or increased energy levels.
3. **Personalize the Program**:
   - Everyone's gut health journey is unique. Tracking enables you to tailor the program to suit your specific needs.
4. **Stay Motivated**:
   - Recording small wins keeps you motivated and focused on your goals, especially during challenging moments.

What to Track

To gain a comprehensive view of your progress, track the following key areas:

1. Symptoms

- **Digestive Symptoms**:
  - Bloating
  - Gas
  - Diarrhea
  - Constipation
  - Acid reflux
- **Other Physical Symptoms**:
  - Skin issues (e.g., acne, eczema)
  - Joint pain or stiffness
  - Food sensitivities

- Sleep quality

2. Mood
- Emotional well-being is closely tied to gut health through the **gut-brain axis**.
  - Anxiety
  - Depression
  - Irritability
  - Brain fog
  - Stress levels

3. Energy Levels
- Measure daily fluctuations in energy:
  - Morning alertness
  - Midday productivity
  - Evening fatigue

4. Diet and Lifestyle Factors
- Foods and beverages consumed.
- Supplements taken (type and dosage).
- Exercise routines and physical activity.
- Stress-management practices (e.g., yoga, meditation).
- Sleep duration and quality.

How to Track Progress

1. Journaling

A dedicated health journal is an excellent way to record and reflect on your progress.

Sections to Include:
- **Daily Log:**
  - Meals and snacks (include portion sizes and any new foods introduced).
  - Symptoms experienced (rate severity on a scale of 1–10).
  - Mood and emotional state.
  - Energy levels (morning, afternoon, evening).
- **Weekly Reflections:**
  - Overall trends (e.g., fewer bloating episodes, improved sleep).
  - New insights or patterns (e.g., "I noticed bloating after

eating dairy-free yogurt").

Example Entry:
- **Date:** January 1, 2024
- **Meals:** Breakfast – Gut-healing smoothie; Lunch – Grilled salmon with broccoli; Dinner – Bone broth soup.
- **Symptoms:** Mild bloating (3/10) after lunch, no constipation.
- **Mood:** Calm and focused in the morning; slight irritability in the evening.
- **Energy Levels:** High in the morning (8/10), moderate in the afternoon (6/10), low in the evening (4/10).

2. Symptom Tracker

A symptom tracker is a quick way to monitor daily changes without detailed journaling. Use a spreadsheet, app, or printable template to record:

- **Date**
- **Severity of Symptoms** (1 = mild, 10 = severe)
    - Bloating
    - Gas
    - Digestive pain
    - Skin flare-ups
    - Fatigue
- **Notes:**
    - Include triggers or context (e.g., "Bloating after eating raw onions").

3. Mood and Energy Rating Scales

Use a simple numerical or color-coded system to track mood and energy:

- **Mood Rating:** 1 = Very low, 10 = Very high.
- **Energy Rating:** 1 = Exhausted, 10 = Energetic.

Example:
- Morning Mood: 7/10
- Midday Energy: 5/10
- Evening Mood: 4/10

4. Food and Symptom Correlation Chart

A correlation chart helps identify specific foods that trigger

symptoms.
- **Column 1**: Food/Beverage Consumed
- **Column 2**: Time of Consumption
- **Column 3**: Symptoms Experienced
- **Column 4**: Time Symptoms Occurred
- **Column 5**: Severity (1–10)

Example:

Food	Time	Symptoms	Onset Time	Severity
Dairy-free yogurt	8:00 AM	Bloating, gas	9:30 AM	4/10
Grilled chicken	12:30 PM	No symptoms	N/A	N/A

5. Photos and Visual Progress

Take photos of your skin, meals, or even posture to visually document improvements:
- **Skin**: If dealing with gut-related acne or eczema, photograph your skin weekly to track visible changes.
- **Meals**: Photograph meals to identify patterns in nutrient diversity.

Tools for Tracking

1. **Apps**:
   - **MyFitnessPal**: Tracks food intake and symptoms.
   - **Cara Care**: Focuses on gut health, allowing you to log symptoms, food, and mood.
   - **Daylio**: Tracks mood and energy levels with a simple interface.
2. **Spreadsheets**:
   - Use Google Sheets or Excel to create a custom tracker.
   - Include columns for symptoms, meals, supplements, and lifestyle factors.
3. **Printable Templates**:

- Use ready-made templates for symptom and mood tracking.

Tips for Effective Tracking
1. **Be Consistent**:
   - Record entries daily, even if only briefly. Consistency is key to spotting trends.
2. **Be Honest**:
   - Don't sugarcoat or omit symptoms. Honest tracking provides the most accurate picture.
3. **Track New Introductions**:
   - When adding new foods or supplements, log their effects over several days to identify positive or negative reactions.
4. **Reflect Weekly**:
   - Review your entries at the end of each week to summarize patterns or improvements.

What to Look for Over 30 Days
- **Digestive Improvements**:
  - Reduced frequency and severity of bloating, gas, or diarrhea.
  - More regular bowel movements.
- **Energy Gains**:
  - Increased energy levels throughout the day.
  - Less afternoon fatigue.
- **Mood Stabilization**:
  - Fewer instances of irritability or anxiety.
  - Improved mental clarity and focus.
- **Symptom Reduction**:
  - Alleviation of skin conditions or joint pain.
  - Improved sleep quality.

When to Adjust Your Program
1. **If Symptoms Persist**:
   - Reevaluate potential irritants in your diet or adjust supplement dosages.
2. **If Energy Remains Low**:

- Consider adding more healthy fats or addressing nutrient deficiencies.
3. **If No Improvements Occur by Week 3:**
    - Consult a healthcare professional for additional testing (e.g., food sensitivities, microbiome analysis).

Chapter 7: Lifestyle Changes to Support Long-Term Gut Health

Achieving a healthy gut goes beyond dietary changes and supplements. Long-term gut health is a result of consistent, sustainable **lifestyle choices** that support the gut-brain axis, promote microbial diversity, and reduce systemic inflammation. This chapter explores lifestyle modifications essential for maintaining a healthy gut and ensuring your digestive system thrives for years to come.

1. Prioritize Stress Management

Chronic stress is a significant contributor to gut health issues, including **leaky gut syndrome, IBS**, and **gut dysbiosis**. When stress activates the **sympathetic nervous system** (fight-or-flight mode), it disrupts digestion, weakens the gut lining, and alters the balance of gut bacteria.

Key Practices for Stress Reduction
- **Meditation:** Spend 10–20 minutes daily practicing mindfulness meditation to calm your mind and body.
- **Yoga:** Incorporate yoga poses like **Child's Pose** or **Supine Twist** to relax the abdominal muscles and stimulate the

parasympathetic nervous system.
- **Deep Breathing Exercises**:
    - Practice **diaphragmatic breathing**, where you inhale deeply through your nose, allowing your belly to expand, and exhale slowly.
    - Aim for 5 minutes twice a day.

Long-Term Tip:

Schedule time daily for activities that reduce stress, whether it's a hobby, time in nature, or simply unplugging from technology.

2. Optimize Sleep Hygiene

Sleep is essential for gut repair and the production of beneficial gut bacteria. Poor sleep can disrupt the gut-brain axis, leading to inflammation and weakened gut lining integrity.

Tips for Better Sleep
- **Establish a Routine**: Go to bed and wake up at the same time daily to regulate your body's circadian rhythm.
- **Create a Sleep-Friendly Environment**:
    - Keep your bedroom cool, dark, and quiet.
    - Use blackout curtains or a white noise machine if necessary.
- **Avoid Stimulants**: Limit caffeine and screen time at least 2–3 hours before bed.
- **Supplements**:
    - Consider **magnesium glycinate** to promote relaxation.
    - Herbal teas like chamomile or valerian root can also aid in sleep.

Long-Term Tip:

Aim for 7–9 hours of quality sleep each night to allow your gut to reset and repair itself.

3. Stay Physically Active

Regular physical activity has a profound impact on gut health. Exercise increases **gut microbial diversity**, enhances digestion, and reduces systemic inflammation. However, avoid overexertion, which can negatively affect the gut.

Best Exercises for Gut Health

- **Moderate-Intensity Cardio:**
  - Activities like walking, swimming, or cycling promote circulation to the digestive organs and support regular bowel movements.
- **Strength Training:**
  - Builds muscle, improves metabolism, and supports gut health through better glucose regulation.
- **Yoga:**
  - Specific poses like **Cat-Cow Pose** and **Seated Forward Fold** massage the digestive organs and alleviate bloating.

Long-Term Tip:
Incorporate at least 150 minutes of moderate exercise per week and vary your workouts to keep your body and microbiome engaged.

4. Cultivate a Gut-Friendly Eating Schedule

The timing of meals and how you eat significantly impact digestion and gut health. Mindless eating or irregular meal patterns can lead to digestive distress.

Healthy Eating Habits
- **Chew Thoroughly:**
  - Proper chewing breaks down food and activates digestive enzymes, reducing the strain on your gut.
- **Eat Slowly:**
  - Avoid rushing meals. Take time to enjoy your food to prevent overeating and bloating.
- **Regular Meal Times:**
  - Stick to consistent eating schedules to align with your body's natural digestive rhythm.
- **Avoid Late-Night Eating:**
  - Finish your last meal at least 2–3 hours before bedtime to give your gut time to rest overnight.

Long-Term Tip:
Practice mindful eating, focusing on the flavors, textures, and sensations of your meals.

5. Limit Toxin Exposure

Environmental toxins, pesticides, and endocrine disruptors can negatively impact gut health by harming the microbiome and increasing inflammation.

Steps to Minimize Toxin Exposure
- **Choose Organic Foods**:
  - Whenever possible, opt for organic produce and meats to reduce pesticide intake.
- **Filter Your Water**:
  - Use a high-quality water filter to remove contaminants like chlorine and heavy metals.
- **Reduce Processed Products**:
  - Avoid foods with artificial additives, preservatives, and emulsifiers that can disrupt gut bacteria.
- **Switch to Non-Toxic Products**:
  - Use eco-friendly cleaning and personal care products free from harmful chemicals.

Long-Term Tip:
Read labels carefully and prioritize natural, minimally processed products in all aspects of your life.

6. Foster Social Connections

Social interactions play a surprising role in gut health. Positive relationships and social activities reduce stress and improve the diversity of gut bacteria.

How to Build Meaningful Connections
- **Spend Time with Loved Ones**:
  - Regularly engage in activities with family and friends that bring you joy.
- **Join Community Groups**:
  - Participate in clubs, fitness classes, or volunteer work to expand your social circle.
- **Practice Gratitude**:
  - Cultivate gratitude to enhance emotional well-being, which indirectly supports gut health.

Long-Term Tip:
Nurture relationships that bring positivity into your life and limit exposure to toxic or stressful interactions.

7. Avoid Overuse of Medications

Certain medications, particularly antibiotics and non-steroidal anti-inflammatory drugs (NSAIDs), can disrupt the gut microbiome and damage the gut lining.

Tips for Responsible Medication Use
- **Antibiotics**: Only use antibiotics when absolutely necessary and always pair them with a high-quality probiotic supplement.
- **NSAIDs**: Limit use of ibuprofen and similar drugs to avoid gut irritation.
- **Proactive Health Care**:
  - Work with a healthcare provider to explore alternative treatments that are gentler on the gut.

Long-Term Tip:
Prioritize preventive care and consult your doctor about gut-friendly alternatives to common medications.

8. Stay Hydrated

Hydration is critical for digestion and gut health. Proper hydration supports the movement of food through the intestines, reduces bloating, and helps maintain the mucosal lining of the gut.

Hydration Tips
- **Drink Enough Water**:
  - Aim for 8–10 glasses of water daily, depending on your activity level and climate.
- **Infused Water**:
  - Add lemon, cucumber, or mint for added flavor and detox benefits.
- **Avoid Sugary Drinks**:
  - Replace sodas and sweetened beverages with herbal teas or plain water.

Long-Term Tip:
Carry a reusable water bottle and make hydration a habit throughout your day.

9. Support Your Gut Microbiome

Maintaining a diverse and balanced gut microbiome is key to long-term gut health.

Practical Strategies
- **Eat a Variety of Foods:**
  - Rotate fruits, vegetables, and proteins to promote microbial diversity.
- **Incorporate Fermented Foods:**
  - Add yogurt, kefir, kimchi, and sauerkraut to your diet for natural probiotics.
- **Add Prebiotics:**
  - Include foods like garlic, onions, asparagus, and bananas to feed beneficial bacteria.

Long-Term Tip:
Focus on a fiber-rich, whole-food diet to nurture your microbiome and avoid over-reliance on supplements.

10. Practice Self-Compassion

Healing and maintaining gut health is a journey. Self-compassion can reduce stress and prevent you from feeling overwhelmed.

Ways to Cultivate Self-Compassion
- **Set Realistic Goals:**
  - Recognize that progress takes time and celebrate small victories.
- **Focus on the Positive:**
  - Acknowledge improvements in your gut health and overall well-being.
- **Forgive Setbacks:**
  - If you deviate from your plan, use it as a learning experience and refocus on your goals.

Sleep and Gut Health: How Proper Sleep Improves Gut Health and Strategies for Better Rest

Sleep and gut health are deeply interconnected. The **gut-brain axis**, a two-way communication system between the brain and gut, plays a crucial role in maintaining optimal health. Poor sleep disrupts this axis, leading to imbalances in the gut microbiome, increased gut permeability, and heightened inflammation. Conversely, a healthy gut promotes restorative sleep by producing neurotransmitters like serotonin and melatonin, which regulate the sleep-wake cycle.

This chapter explores how proper sleep supports gut health, the consequences of inadequate rest, and actionable strategies to improve sleep quality for enhanced gut healing and overall well-being.

1. The Connection Between Sleep and Gut Health

How Sleep Impacts the Gut

1. **Microbial Balance:**
   - Sleep influences the composition and diversity of the **gut microbiome**. Poor sleep can disrupt microbial balance, leading to gut dysbiosis (an imbalance of harmful and beneficial bacteria).
   - Dysbiosis has been linked to digestive issues, leaky gut, and inflammation.

2. **Intestinal Barrier Function:**
   - During sleep, the body repairs the **intestinal lining**, reducing gut permeability. Sleep deprivation hinders this repair process, increasing the risk of leaky gut.

3. **Inflammation:**
   - Lack of sleep increases the production of pro-inflammatory cytokines, which can damage the gut lining and worsen chronic conditions like IBS or autoimmune diseases.

4. **Hormonal Regulation:**
   - Sleep regulates cortisol, the stress hormone. High cortisol levels caused by sleep deprivation disrupt digestion, slow gut motility, and weaken the gut lining.

How the Gut Impacts Sleep

1. **Neurotransmitter Production:**
   - The gut produces **serotonin**, a precursor to melatonin, the sleep hormone. A healthy gut ensures adequate melatonin production for restful sleep.

2. **Inflammation and Sleep Disruption:**
   - Gut inflammation can lead to restless sleep and insomnia due to its effects on the nervous system.

2. The Consequences of Poor Sleep on Gut Health

- **Reduced Microbial Diversity:**

- Sleep deprivation decreases beneficial bacteria like **Lactobacillus** and **Bifidobacterium**, which support digestion and immunity.
- **Increased Risk of Digestive Issues**:
  - Poor sleep contributes to bloating, gas, and irregular bowel movements.
- **Worsened Chronic Conditions**:
  - Sleep deprivation exacerbates symptoms of leaky gut, IBS, and autoimmune conditions by increasing inflammation and weakening the immune system.
- **Mood and Gut Connection**:
  - Sleep disruption can worsen anxiety and depression, both of which negatively impact gut health through the gut-brain axis.

3. How Proper Sleep Improves Gut Health

1. **Enhances Microbial Health**:
   - Restorative sleep promotes microbial diversity, fostering a balanced gut environment.
2. **Supports Gut Lining Repair**:
   - Sleep allows for cellular repair and regeneration of the intestinal lining, reducing gut permeability.
3. **Regulates Appetite and Cravings**:
   - Adequate sleep balances hunger hormones like ghrelin and leptin, preventing overconsumption of inflammatory foods.
4. **Reduces Inflammation**:
   - Proper sleep lowers systemic inflammation, protecting the gut lining and promoting better digestion.
5. **Boosts Immunity**:
   - Sleep strengthens the immune system, which is closely tied to gut health.

4. Strategies for Better Sleep to Support Gut Health

a. Create a Sleep-Friendly Environment

1. **Darkness**:
   - Use blackout curtains or an eye mask to eliminate light,

which disrupts melatonin production.
2. **Quietness**:
   - Reduce noise with earplugs or a white noise machine to create a calming atmosphere.
3. **Temperature**:
   - Keep the bedroom cool (60–67°F or 15–19°C) to support deep sleep.

b. Maintain a Consistent Sleep Schedule
- **Wake and Sleep Times**:
   - Go to bed and wake up at the same time every day, even on weekends, to regulate your circadian rhythm.
- **Pre-Bedtime Routine**:
   - Establish a relaxing routine, such as reading, meditation, or a warm bath, to signal your body that it's time to wind down.

c. Avoid Sleep Disruptors
1. **Blue Light**:
   - Limit screen time (TV, phones, tablets) at least 2–3 hours before bed. Blue light suppresses melatonin production.
2. **Caffeine**:
   - Avoid caffeine after 2 PM, as it can interfere with falling asleep.
3. **Alcohol**:
   - Limit alcohol consumption, which disrupts sleep quality and REM cycles.

d. Incorporate Relaxation Techniques
1. **Meditation**:
   - Practice mindfulness or guided meditation to calm the mind and reduce cortisol levels.
2. **Deep Breathing**:
   - Perform diaphragmatic breathing exercises to activate the parasympathetic nervous system.
3. **Progressive Muscle Relaxation**:
   - Tense and release each muscle group to reduce physical tension and promote relaxation.

e. Optimize Your Diet for Better Sleep
1. **Melatonin-Rich Foods**:
   - Include cherries, walnuts, and tomatoes to support natural melatonin production.
2. **Magnesium-Rich Foods**:
   - Eat leafy greens, almonds, and bananas to promote muscle relaxation and calmness.
3. **Prebiotic Foods**:
   - Incorporate foods like garlic, onions, and asparagus to nourish gut bacteria and improve sleep via the gut-brain axis.
4. **Light Evening Meals**:
   - Avoid heavy, rich foods close to bedtime, which can disrupt digestion and sleep.

f. Consider Supplements
1. **Magnesium Glycinate**:
   - Supports relaxation and better sleep quality.
2. **Melatonin**:
   - Aids in resetting your circadian rhythm, especially during periods of sleep disruption.
3. **Probiotics**:
   - Improves microbial health, which indirectly supports melatonin and serotonin production.
4. **L-Theanine**:
   - A calming amino acid that reduces anxiety and promotes relaxation.

g. Get Morning Sunlight
- Exposure to natural light in the morning helps regulate your circadian rhythm by signaling your body to produce cortisol during the day and melatonin at night.

5. Tracking Sleep and Gut Progress
1. **Sleep Journals**:
   - Record sleep duration, quality, and any disturbances.
2. **Symptom Tracking**:
   - Note changes in gut symptoms (bloating, digestion,

bowel movements) relative to sleep quality.
3. **Sleep Apps**:
    - Use apps like **Sleep Cycle** or **Fitbit** to monitor sleep patterns and improvements.

6. Combining Sleep and Gut Health Practices

For maximum benefits, integrate sleep strategies with gut-friendly practices:
- Follow an **anti-inflammatory diet** during the day.
- Incorporate **gentle evening yoga** to relax the body.
- Take **probiotics and prebiotics** to support microbial health, which will improve your sleep-wake cycle over time.

Exercise and Movement: The Role of Physical Activity in Supporting Gut Health and the Best Types of Exercise for Women

Physical activity is an essential component of gut health. Regular exercise improves digestion, enhances microbial diversity, reduces inflammation, and supports the overall health of the **gut-brain axis**. For women, incorporating movement into daily life can also address unique challenges like hormonal fluctuations, stress, and bone health, all of which influence gut function.

In this chapter, we'll explore the connection between exercise and gut health, the benefits of physical activity for women, and the best types of exercise to include in a gut-supportive routine.

1. The Connection Between Exercise and Gut Health

a. Improves Microbial Diversity
- Regular exercise has been shown to **increase the diversity of gut bacteria**, which is critical for a healthy microbiome. A diverse microbiome enhances digestion, immune function, and mood regulation.
- Active individuals tend to have higher levels of **beneficial bacteria** like *Akkermansia muciniphila* and *Bifidobacterium*, which protect the gut lining and reduce inflammation.

b. Reduces Gut Inflammation
- Exercise lowers the production of pro-inflammatory cytokines, reducing gut-related inflammation and supporting conditions like **IBS** and **leaky gut syndrome**.

c. Enhances Gut Motility
- Physical activity stimulates the **muscles of the digestive tract**, promoting regular bowel movements and preventing constipation.
- Aerobic exercises, in particular, improve blood flow to the gut, aiding digestion and nutrient absorption.

d. Regulates the Gut-Brain Axis
- Exercise reduces stress and improves mood by lowering cortisol levels and increasing the production of **serotonin**—a neurotransmitter largely produced in the gut.
- A calmer nervous system translates to better gut function and fewer stress-related digestive issues.

2. Benefits of Exercise for Women's Gut Health

a. Hormonal Balance
- Exercise helps regulate **estrogen** and **progesterone**, hormones that influence gut motility and microbiome composition. Hormonal fluctuations during menstruation, pregnancy, or menopause can disrupt gut health, but regular movement mitigates these effects.

b. Bone Health and Digestion
- Weight-bearing exercises improve bone density while supporting the digestive system by stimulating the core muscles, which aids gut motility.

c. Stress Reduction
- Women often experience high levels of chronic stress due to busy schedules and multiple responsibilities. Stress impacts the gut through increased cortisol, but regular exercise lowers stress hormones, supporting gut health.

d. Pelvic Floor Strength
- Strengthening the pelvic floor improves gut health by promoting proper posture, which aids in digestion, and preventing issues like constipation or bloating.

3. The Best Types of Exercise for Gut Health

a. Low-Impact Aerobic Exercise
- **Examples**: Walking, swimming, cycling.

- **Benefits**:
  - Increases heart rate, which boosts circulation to the digestive organs.
  - Gentle on the joints, making it suitable for women of all fitness levels.
  - Reduces bloating and promotes regular bowel movements.

b. Strength Training
- **Examples**: Weight lifting, resistance band exercises, bodyweight exercises (e.g., squats, lunges).
- **Benefits**:
  - Builds muscle and improves metabolism, which supports overall gut health.
  - Encourages the release of endorphins, reducing stress.
  - Enhances core strength, aiding in better digestion.

c. Yoga
- **Examples**: Gentle yoga flows, restorative yoga, or specific gut-supportive poses.
- **Benefits**:
  - Improves gut motility and reduces stress through deep breathing and stretching.
  - Specific poses like **Seated Twist**, **Child's Pose**, and **Cat-Cow** massage the digestive organs, alleviating bloating and constipation.
  - Activates the parasympathetic nervous system (rest-and-digest mode).

d. Pilates
- Focuses on strengthening the core and pelvic floor, which enhances gut function and prevents issues like constipation.
- Improves posture, which reduces pressure on the abdomen and supports digestion.

e. High-Intensity Interval Training (HIIT)
- **Examples**: Short bursts of cardio followed by rest periods, such as cycling or jumping jacks.
- **Benefits**:

- Boosts metabolism and promotes the growth of beneficial gut bacteria.
- Efficient for women with busy schedules, as it delivers benefits in a shorter time frame.

f. Mindful Movement
- **Examples**: Tai chi, Qigong.
- **Benefits**:
  - Combines slow, intentional movements with breath control to reduce stress and improve digestion.
  - Enhances the mind-body connection, supporting the gut-brain axis.

4. Creating a Gut-Friendly Exercise Routine

a. Frequency
- Aim for at least **150 minutes of moderate-intensity exercise** per week.
- Incorporate a mix of aerobic, strength, and flexibility exercises for balanced benefits.

b. Timing
- **Morning**: Start the day with light aerobic exercise like walking or yoga to stimulate digestion.
- **Post-Meals**: A short walk after meals can reduce bloating and aid digestion.
- **Evening**: Gentle exercises like restorative yoga promote relaxation and better sleep.

c. Intensity
- Avoid overexertion, as intense exercise can increase cortisol levels, which may disrupt gut health.
- Focus on moderate-intensity activities that are sustainable and enjoyable.

5. Tips for Supporting Gut Health Through Exercise

1. **Stay Hydrated**:
   - Drink water before, during, and after exercise to support digestion and prevent dehydration.
2. **Listen to Your Body**:
   - Avoid exercising immediately after a large meal, as this

can disrupt digestion. Wait at least 1–2 hours.
3. **Warm-Up and Cool Down**:
   - Gentle stretches before and after workouts prevent muscle strain and aid circulation to the gut.
4. **Incorporate Core Work**:
   - Strengthen your core muscles with exercises like planks and leg raises to support gut motility.
5. **Pair Movement with Breathwork**:
   - Focus on deep, diaphragmatic breathing during workouts to calm the nervous system and optimize gut-brain communication.

6. Monitoring Progress

Track how exercise impacts your gut health by:
- Keeping a **symptom journal** to note improvements in digestion, energy levels, and mood.
- Monitoring changes in bowel regularity and bloating.

Stress Management: Techniques to Prevent Gut Flare-Ups

Stress has a profound impact on gut health. The **gut-brain axis**, a bi-directional communication system between the gut and brain, means that stress in the mind translates to disturbances in the digestive system. Chronic stress can weaken the gut lining, disrupt the gut microbiome, and trigger conditions like **leaky gut**, **IBS**, and **inflammation**. Managing daily stress effectively is essential for preventing gut flare-ups and promoting long-term digestive health.

This chapter explores stress management techniques such as mindfulness, breathing exercises, and strategies for reducing daily stress to support gut healing and overall well-being.

1. How Stress Affects Gut Health

a. The Gut-Brain Axis
- Stress activates the **sympathetic nervous system** (fight-or-flight mode), reducing blood flow to the digestive organs and impairing digestion.
- Chronic stress elevates cortisol levels, which disrupts gut motility, weakens the intestinal barrier, and promotes inflammation.

b. Gut Microbiome Imbalance
- Stress alters the composition and diversity of the **gut microbiome**, reducing beneficial bacteria and increasing harmful strains.
- This imbalance can lead to symptoms such as bloating, gas, and irregular bowel movements.

c. Inflammation
- Prolonged stress triggers systemic inflammation, exacerbating gut conditions like **IBD** and **leaky gut syndrome**.

2. Mindfulness Practices for Gut Health

Mindfulness is the practice of being fully present and aware of the moment without judgment. It has been shown to reduce stress, improve digestion, and support gut healing by activating the **parasympathetic nervous system** (rest-and-digest mode).

a. Mindful Meditation
- **What It Is**: A practice of sitting quietly and focusing on your breath or a mantra.
- **How It Helps**:
    - Lowers cortisol levels.
    - Enhances the gut-brain connection by promoting relaxation.
- **How to Practice**:
    - Find a quiet, comfortable space.
    - Close your eyes and take slow, deep breaths.
    - Focus on your breath, a word, or a phrase (e.g., "calm" or "peace").
    - Start with 5–10 minutes daily, gradually increasing to 20 minutes.

b. Mindful Eating
- **What It Is**: Paying full attention to your meals, including the taste, texture, and sensations of eating.
- **How It Helps**:
    - Promotes better digestion by reducing stress while eating.
    - Prevents overeating and reduces bloating.
- **How to Practice**:

- Turn off distractions like TV or smartphones.
- Take small bites and chew slowly.
- Focus on the flavors, textures, and aromas of your food.

c. Gratitude Journaling
- **What It Is**: Writing down things you're grateful for daily.
- **How It Helps**:
  - Shifts focus away from stressors, reducing their impact on gut health.
- **How to Practice**:
  - Spend 5 minutes at the end of each day writing down 3–5 things you're grateful for.
  - Reflect on positive moments or accomplishments.

3. Breathing Exercises for Stress Reduction
Deep breathing is one of the simplest and most effective tools for calming the nervous system and preventing gut flare-ups.

a. Diaphragmatic Breathing
- **What It Is**: A deep breathing technique that engages the diaphragm, expanding the belly rather than the chest.
- **How It Helps**:
  - Activates the parasympathetic nervous system.
  - Increases oxygen flow to the gut, supporting digestion.
- **How to Practice**:
  - Sit or lie down in a comfortable position.
  - Place one hand on your chest and the other on your belly.
  - Inhale deeply through your nose, allowing your belly to rise.
  - Exhale slowly through your mouth, letting your belly fall.
  - Repeat for 5–10 minutes.

b. Box Breathing
- **What It Is**: A structured breathing exercise used to reduce anxiety and calm the mind.
- **How It Helps**:
  - Lowers heart rate and cortisol levels.
  - Improves focus and reduces gut-related stress symptoms.
- **How to Practice**:

- Inhale through your nose for 4 counts.
- Hold your breath for 4 counts.
- Exhale through your mouth for 4 counts.
- Hold your breath for 4 counts.
- Repeat for 3–5 minutes.

c. **Alternate Nostril Breathing (Nadi Shodhana)**
- **What It Is**: A yogic breathing practice that balances the nervous system.
- **How It Helps**:
  - Promotes relaxation and reduces stress.
  - Enhances focus and clarity.
- **How to Practice**:
  - Sit comfortably and close your right nostril with your thumb.
  - Inhale through your left nostril.
  - Close your left nostril with your ring finger and release your thumb from the right nostril.
  - Exhale through the right nostril.
  - Repeat, alternating nostrils for 5 minutes.

4. Managing Daily Stress to Prevent Gut Flare-Ups

Stress is an inevitable part of life, but managing it effectively can prevent it from harming your gut.

a. **Time Management**
- **Prioritize Tasks**:
  - Use tools like to-do lists or planners to organize your day.
  - Break large tasks into smaller, manageable steps.
- **Set Boundaries**:
  - Learn to say no to unnecessary commitments to avoid burnout.

b. **Physical Activity**
- Regular exercise lowers stress levels and supports gut health. Low-impact activities like yoga, walking, or swimming are particularly effective.

c. **Social Connection**
- **How It Helps**:

- Positive relationships reduce stress and support emotional well-being.
- **How to Practice**:
  - Spend time with friends and family regularly.
  - Join community groups or engage in hobbies that connect you with others.

d. Digital Detox
- **How It Helps**:
  - Reducing screen time lowers cortisol levels and prevents overstimulation.
- **How to Practice**:
  - Set specific times to unplug from digital devices.
  - Avoid screens at least 1–2 hours before bedtime to improve sleep.

5. Evening Rituals to Wind Down

Establishing a calming evening routine can help you manage stress and improve gut health.

a. Herbal Teas
- **Chamomile or Peppermint Tea**:
  - Soothes the digestive system and promotes relaxation.

b. Gentle Yoga
- Poses like **Child's Pose** or **Supine Twist** relieve tension in the abdomen and calm the nervous system.

c. Journaling
- Write down any worries or tasks for the next day to clear your mind before sleep.

6. Monitoring Progress

Track how stress management impacts your gut health by:
- **Journaling Symptoms**:
  - Record instances of bloating, discomfort, or irregular bowel movements.
  - Note if symptoms correlate with high-stress days.
- **Mood Tracking**:
  - Reflect on emotional well-being and how stress management practices make you feel.

- **Sleep Quality**:
    - Observe improvements in sleep patterns, which indicate reduced stress.

Toxin-Free Living: Minimizing Exposure to Environmental Toxins That Impact Gut Health

Environmental toxins play a significant but often overlooked role in gut health. Many common household products, personal care items, and even the foods we consume contain chemicals that can disrupt the gut microbiome, damage the intestinal lining, and increase inflammation. Adopting a toxin-free lifestyle is a proactive way to protect your gut, improve overall health, and reduce the burden on your body's natural detoxification systems.

This chapter provides practical advice on minimizing toxin exposure, focusing on areas like cleaning products, personal care, food, water, and home environment.

1. How Environmental Toxins Affect Gut Health
a. Disruption of the Gut Microbiome
- Chemicals like pesticides, BPA, and phthalates disrupt the balance of gut bacteria, reducing the diversity of beneficial microbes and promoting the growth of harmful strains.

b. Damage to the Gut Lining
- Certain toxins weaken the gut lining, increasing **intestinal permeability** (leaky gut), which allows harmful substances to enter the bloodstream and trigger inflammation.

c. Inflammation
- Exposure to environmental toxins elevates systemic inflammation, exacerbating gut-related issues such as **IBS**, **autoimmune diseases**, and **chronic fatigue**.

d. Hormonal Disruption
- Endocrine-disrupting chemicals (EDCs) like BPA and parabens interfere with hormone regulation, indirectly impacting gut motility and microbiome balance.

2. Toxin-Free Cleaning Products
Many conventional cleaning products contain harsh chemicals like ammonia, bleach, and synthetic fragrances, which can release volatile

organic compounds (VOCs) that harm both the gut and respiratory systems.

Switch to Non-Toxic Cleaning Alternatives
- **All-Purpose Cleaner:**
  - Use a mix of **white vinegar** and **water** (1:1 ratio) with a few drops of essential oils (e.g., lemon or tea tree) for antibacterial properties.
- **Glass Cleaner:**
  - Combine water, white vinegar, and a teaspoon of cornstarch for streak-free windows.
- **Laundry Detergent:**
  - Choose biodegradable, fragrance-free detergents with natural ingredients like **soap nuts** or plant-based surfactants.

Avoid These Ingredients:
- Ammonia
- Bleach
- Triclosan
- Synthetic fragrances
- Formaldehyde-releasing agents

Practical Tips:
- Check labels for certifications like **EPA Safer Choice**, **ECOLOGO**, or **Green Seal**.
- Reduce airborne toxins by ventilating your home during and after cleaning.

3. Non-Toxic Personal Care Products
Personal care products like shampoos, lotions, and cosmetics often contain harmful chemicals that are absorbed through the skin and can disrupt gut health indirectly.

Key Ingredients to Avoid:
- **Parabens:** Linked to hormonal disruption.
- **Phthalates:** Found in fragrances, disrupt gut microbiota and hormones.
- **Sodium Lauryl Sulfate (SLS):** Irritates the skin and may trigger inflammation.

- **BHA/BHT**: Artificial preservatives harmful to the gut and liver.

Switch to Safer Alternatives:
- **Shampoos and Conditioners**:
  - Look for sulfate-free and paraben-free options made with natural oils and botanical extracts.
- **Toothpaste**:
  - Choose fluoride-free toothpaste without triclosan.
- **Deodorants**:
  - Opt for aluminum-free, fragrance-free formulas made with baking soda or magnesium.
- **Cosmetics**:
  - Seek products with **non-toxic certifications** such as **EWG Verified** or **COSMOS Organic**.

DIY Personal Care:
- Make a simple face scrub using **coconut oil** and **sugar**.
- Use **aloe vera gel** as a moisturizer for a toxin-free alternative.

4. Minimize Toxins in Food

What we eat is a major source of exposure to pesticides, preservatives, and artificial additives that harm gut health.

Choose Organic and Non-GMO:
- Prioritize organic produce to reduce exposure to pesticides like glyphosate, which disrupts gut bacteria.
- Use the **EWG Dirty Dozen** and **Clean Fifteen** lists to decide which produce to buy organic.

Avoid Processed Foods:
- Cut back on foods containing artificial colors, flavors, and preservatives.
- Eliminate foods with emulsifiers like carrageenan and polysorbates, which can damage the gut lining.

Store Food Safely:
- Avoid plastic containers with **BPA** or **phthalates**; use glass, stainless steel, or silicone alternatives.
- Never microwave food in plastic containers.

Wash Produce Thoroughly:
- Use a homemade produce wash:

- Combine 1 part vinegar with 3 parts water to soak fruits and vegetables for 5–10 minutes, then rinse.

5. Drink Clean, Filtered Water

Tap water can contain chlorine, fluoride, heavy metals, and other contaminants that disrupt gut health.

Use a Water Filtration System:
- **Carbon Filters**: Remove chlorine, VOCs, and sediment.
- **Reverse Osmosis**: Provides a higher level of filtration, removing fluoride and heavy metals.

Practical Tips:
- Replace bottled water with reusable bottles made of stainless steel or glass to avoid leaching from plastic.

6. Improve Indoor Air Quality

Indoor air is often more polluted than outdoor air due to VOCs, mold, and dust, which can affect gut health indirectly.

Reduce Airborne Toxins:
- Use a HEPA air purifier to remove dust, allergens, and airborne chemicals.
- Incorporate **houseplants** like spider plants, snake plants, or peace lilies, which filter indoor air.

Avoid Synthetic Air Fresheners:
- Replace with natural alternatives like **essential oil diffusers** or dried herbs (e.g., lavender sachets).

Control Mold:
- Address leaks or dampness promptly, as mold spores can trigger inflammation and weaken gut health.

7. Minimize Exposure to Endocrine Disruptors

Endocrine-disrupting chemicals (EDCs) harm gut health by interfering with hormones that regulate digestion and microbial balance.

Avoid Plastics:
- Choose **BPA-free** or **phthalate-free** products.
- Switch to glass containers for food storage.

Be Cautious with Cans:
- Many canned goods are lined with BPA-containing materials; opt for **BPA-free cans** or fresh alternatives.

Use Safer Cookware:
- Avoid non-stick cookware containing **PFAS** (per- and polyfluoroalkyl substances). Use stainless steel, cast iron, or ceramic cookware instead.

8. Create a Toxin-Free Sleep Environment
Sleep is crucial for gut repair, but a toxin-laden bedroom can disrupt both sleep and gut health.

Replace Toxic Bedding:
- Use organic cotton or bamboo sheets free from synthetic dyes and formaldehyde.

Mattresses:
- Avoid mattresses treated with flame retardants; look for **GREENGUARD-certified** or organic options.

Dust-Free Environment:
- Vacuum and dust regularly to remove allergens and pollutants.

9. Detox Your Daily Routine
Small changes can significantly reduce your overall toxic load:
- **Minimize Chemical Exposure at Work:**
  - Avoid handling receipts coated with **BPA/BPS**.
- **Be Mindful of Pest Control:**
  - Use natural solutions like diatomaceous earth or boric acid instead of chemical pesticides.

10. Practical Steps to Get Started
1. **Gradual Transition:**
   - Replace one product at a time as you run out to make the switch manageable and budget-friendly.
2. **Read Labels:**
   - Learn to identify harmful ingredients and choose safer alternatives.
3. **Invest in Key Areas:**
   - Focus on high-impact changes like water filtration, organic produce, and safer cleaning products.
4. **Stay Informed:**
   - Use resources like the **Environmental Working Group (EWG)** to research product safety.

Toxin-Free Living: Practical Advice on Minimizing Exposure to Environmental Toxins That Impact Gut Health

Environmental toxins are pervasive in modern life, found in everything from household cleaning supplies to the food we eat. These toxins can negatively impact gut health by altering the gut microbiome, increasing intestinal permeability (leaky gut), and triggering chronic inflammation. Transitioning to toxin-free living is a proactive way to protect your gut and improve overall well-being.

This chapter provides **practical advice** on minimizing exposure to environmental toxins, with a focus on cleaning products, food, personal care items, and more. By adopting these strategies, you can create a healthier environment that supports gut health.

1. How Environmental Toxins Impact Gut Health

a. Disruption of the Gut Microbiome
- Chemicals such as **pesticides**, **BPA**, and **phthalates** disturb the balance of beneficial gut bacteria, leading to dysbiosis.
- A disrupted microbiome can contribute to digestive disorders, weakened immunity, and mood disturbances.

b. Damage to the Gut Lining
- Toxins can weaken the intestinal barrier, increasing **intestinal permeability**, also known as leaky gut. This allows harmful substances to enter the bloodstream, triggering inflammation and autoimmune responses.

c. Systemic Inflammation
- Exposure to environmental toxins promotes chronic inflammation, which exacerbates gut-related conditions like **IBD**, **IBS**, and **leaky gut syndrome**.

d. Hormonal Interference
- Many toxins act as **endocrine disruptors**, interfering with hormones that regulate digestion and gut motility.

2. Transitioning to Non-Toxic Cleaning Products

Many conventional cleaning products contain harmful chemicals such as **bleach**, **ammonia**, and **synthetic fragrances**, which release volatile organic compounds (VOCs) into the air. These compounds can be absorbed through inhalation and contact, negatively affecting the gut and

overall health.
Non-Toxic Cleaning Alternatives
1. **All-Purpose Cleaner:**
    - DIY Solution: Mix equal parts white vinegar and water with a few drops of essential oil (e.g., tea tree or lavender) for an effective, antibacterial cleaner.
    - Store-Bought: Look for products certified by **EPA Safer Choice**, **ECOLOGO**, or **Green Seal**.
2. **Glass Cleaner:**
    - DIY Solution: Combine 1 cup water, 1 cup vinegar, and 1 teaspoon cornstarch for streak-free windows.
3. **Laundry Detergent:**
    - Opt for biodegradable detergents free from synthetic fragrances, dyes, and phosphates.
    - Natural alternatives: **Soap nuts** or detergents made from plant-based surfactants.
4. **Air Fresheners:**
    - Avoid synthetic sprays and opt for natural options like essential oil diffusers, potpourri, or baking soda to neutralize odors.

Ingredients to Avoid
- Ammonia
- Chlorine bleach
- Triclosan
- Synthetic fragrances
- Phthalates
- Formaldehyde

3. Reducing Toxins in Food
Food is a significant source of exposure to pesticides, preservatives, and other harmful additives that can harm the gut.

a. Choose Organic and Non-GMO Foods
- Organic produce is grown without synthetic pesticides like **glyphosate**, which disrupts gut bacteria.
- Prioritize buying organic for items on the **EWG Dirty Dozen** list (e.g., strawberries, spinach, apples).

- Look for **Non-GMO Project Verified** labels to avoid genetically modified ingredients that may disrupt gut health.

b. Avoid Processed Foods
- Processed foods often contain:
    - **Artificial additives** (colors, flavors, and preservatives).
    - **Emulsifiers** (e.g., carrageenan, polysorbates), which can damage the gut lining.
    - **Refined sugars**, which feed harmful gut bacteria.
- Opt for whole, minimally processed foods.

c. Store Food Safely
- Replace plastic containers with **glass, stainless steel**, or **silicone** to avoid exposure to BPA and phthalates.
- Avoid microwaving food in plastic containers, as heat increases chemical leaching.

d. Wash Produce Thoroughly
- DIY Produce Wash: Mix 1 part white vinegar with 3 parts water to soak fruits and vegetables for 10 minutes before rinsing.

4. Switching to Non-Toxic Personal Care Products

Personal care products like shampoos, lotions, and makeup often contain harmful chemicals that can be absorbed through the skin and indirectly affect gut health.

Key Ingredients to Avoid
- **Parabens**: Act as endocrine disruptors, affecting hormonal balance and digestion.
- **Phthalates**: Found in synthetic fragrances, linked to microbiome disruption.
- **Sodium Lauryl Sulfate (SLS)**: Can irritate the skin and promote inflammation.
- **BHA/BHT**: Synthetic preservatives harmful to the gut and liver.

Safer Alternatives
1. **Shampoo and Conditioner**:
    - Choose sulfate-free and paraben-free options made with natural ingredients.
2. **Toothpaste**:

- Opt for fluoride-free toothpaste without triclosan.
3. **Deodorant:**
    - Use aluminum-free formulas made with baking soda or magnesium.
4. **Makeup:**
    - Look for products labeled **EWG Verified** or **COSMOS Organic**.

DIY Personal Care Ideas
- **Face Scrub**: Combine coconut oil and sugar for a gentle exfoliant.
- **Moisturizer**: Use pure aloe vera gel or shea butter.

5. Filter Your Water
Tap water often contains chlorine, fluoride, heavy metals, and other contaminants that can disrupt the gut microbiome and overall health.

Water Filtration Options
1. **Carbon Filters:**
    - Affordable and effective for removing chlorine and sediment.
2. **Reverse Osmosis Systems:**
    - Removes a wide range of contaminants, including fluoride, heavy metals, and VOCs.
3. **Water Pitchers:**
    - A budget-friendly option for improving water quality at the point of use.

Practical Tips
- Carry a reusable water bottle made of stainless steel or glass to avoid plastic exposure.

6. Improving Indoor Air Quality
Indoor air is often more polluted than outdoor air, with toxins from cleaning products, furniture, and building materials.

Ways to Reduce Airborne Toxins
- **Air Purifiers:**
    - Use HEPA filters to capture dust, mold, and chemical pollutants.
- **Houseplants:**

- Add air-purifying plants like spider plants, snake plants, or peace lilies.
- **Ventilation**:
  - Open windows regularly to improve air circulation.
- **Natural Air Fresheners**:
  - Replace synthetic sprays with essential oil diffusers or natural candles.

7. Detox Your Home Environment

a. Replace Toxic Cookware

- Avoid non-stick cookware containing **PFAS** (per- and polyfluoroalkyl substances).
- Use **stainless steel, cast iron**, or **ceramic** cookware.

b. Choose Safer Furniture

- Look for flame-retardant-free furniture and mattresses labeled **GREENGUARD Certified or CertiPUR-US**.

c. Avoid Harmful Pest Control Products

- Replace chemical pesticides with natural alternatives like diatomaceous earth or essential oil-based sprays.

8. Practical Tips for Transitioning to Toxin-Free Living

a. Gradual Changes

- Start small by replacing one product at a time as it runs out.
- Focus on high-impact areas like cleaning products, food, and water first.

b. Learn to Read Labels

- Avoid products with lengthy, unpronounceable ingredient lists.
- Look for certifications like **USDA Organic, EWG Verified**, or **Made Safe**.

c. DIY Alternatives

- Make your own non-toxic cleaners, skincare, and personal care items using simple ingredients like vinegar, baking soda, and essential oils.

d. Invest in Key Areas

- Prioritize high-impact investments like a water filter, non-toxic cookware, and organic produce.

Chapter 8: Beyond Leaky Gut: Supporting Hormonal Balance and Overall Wellness

Healing **leaky gut** is an essential step toward achieving optimal health, but true wellness extends beyond gut repair. The gut is intricately connected to other systems in the body, particularly hormones. Hormonal imbalances, such as fluctuations in **estrogen, progesterone, cortisol,** and **thyroid hormones**, can negatively impact gut health and vice versa. By addressing these connections, you can not only maintain a strong gut lining but also support hormonal balance and overall wellness.

This chapter delves into the gut-hormone connection and offers practical strategies to support hormonal harmony and long-term health.

1. The Gut-Hormone Connection

Hormones are chemical messengers that regulate processes such as metabolism, mood, reproduction, and digestion. The gut plays a significant role in hormone regulation through its influence on **hormonal production, detoxification,** and the gut-brain axis.

a. Gut Microbiome and Hormones

- The gut microbiome produces and regulates hormones such as

serotonin (affecting mood and sleep) and **ghrelin** (controlling appetite).
- **Estrobolome**, a subset of gut bacteria, metabolizes estrogen. Dysbiosis (imbalance in gut bacteria) can lead to estrogen dominance, affecting menstrual cycles and increasing the risk of hormonal disorders.

b. Leaky Gut and Hormonal Imbalance
- A damaged gut lining allows toxins and undigested particles to enter the bloodstream, triggering inflammation.
- Chronic inflammation disrupts the endocrine system, contributing to conditions like **PCOS, endometriosis**, and **thyroid dysfunction**.

c. Stress Hormones and the Gut
- Chronic stress increases **cortisol**, which negatively impacts the gut by slowing digestion, altering microbiome balance, and weakening the intestinal barrier.

2. Key Hormones Affected by Gut Health

a. Estrogen
- Estrogen dominance occurs when the body has excess estrogen relative to progesterone. This imbalance can lead to bloating, mood swings, irregular periods, and an increased risk of endometriosis.
- Poor gut health hinders the detoxification of estrogen, leading to reabsorption into the bloodstream.

b. Cortisol
- Elevated cortisol levels from chronic stress impair the gut lining and alter microbial diversity.
- A dysregulated cortisol cycle can exacerbate fatigue, cravings, and digestive issues.

c. Thyroid Hormones
- A healthy gut is crucial for **thyroid hormone conversion** (T4 to T3). Dysbiosis and leaky gut can contribute to hypothyroidism or Hashimoto's thyroiditis.

d. Insulin
- Gut health influences insulin sensitivity. Dysbiosis can lead to

blood sugar imbalances, increasing the risk of insulin resistance and weight gain.

3. Strategies to Support Hormonal Balance and Wellness

a. Nourish with Hormone-Balancing Foods

1. **Healthy Fats:**
   - **Sources**: Avocados, olive oil, nuts, seeds, and wild-caught fish.
   - **Benefits**: Support hormone production and reduce inflammation.
2. **Fiber-Rich Foods:**
   - **Sources**: Vegetables, fruits, flaxseeds, and whole grains.
   - **Benefits**: Aid in estrogen detoxification and nourish gut bacteria.
3. **Cruciferous Vegetables**:
   - **Sources**: Broccoli, cauliflower, kale, and Brussels sprouts.
   - **Benefits**: Contain compounds that help detoxify excess estrogen.
4. **Probiotic-Rich Foods:**
   - **Sources**: Yogurt, kefir, sauerkraut, kimchi, and miso.
   - **Benefits**: Promote microbial diversity and gut health.
5. **Magnesium-Rich Foods**:
   - **Sources**: Leafy greens, dark chocolate, nuts, and seeds.
   - **Benefits**: Regulate cortisol and improve sleep quality.

b. Balance Blood Sugar Levels

- **Eat Balanced Meals**: Include protein, healthy fats, and fiber with every meal to prevent blood sugar spikes.
- **Avoid Refined Carbohydrates**: Minimize intake of processed sugars and flours, which can disrupt insulin levels and gut health.
- **Time Meals Strategically**: Eat smaller, frequent meals if needed to avoid blood sugar crashes.

c. Manage Stress Effectively

Chronic stress disrupts the gut-brain axis and contributes to hormonal imbalances. Implement daily stress-reduction techniques:

- **Mindfulness Meditation**: Spend 10–15 minutes daily focusing

on your breath or guided meditations to calm the mind and lower cortisol.
- **Breathwork**: Practice deep breathing exercises to activate the parasympathetic nervous system.
- **Journaling**: Reflect on your stressors and gratitude to process emotions healthily.

d. Prioritize Sleep
Quality sleep is essential for hormonal balance and gut health.
- **Maintain a Consistent Schedule**: Go to bed and wake up at the same time daily.
- **Create a Sleep-Friendly Environment**: Keep your bedroom cool, dark, and free from electronics.
- **Wind Down Naturally**: Avoid caffeine and screen time at least 2 hours before bed.

e. Optimize Detox Pathways
The liver and gut work together to detoxify hormones like estrogen. Support these pathways to maintain hormonal balance.
1. **Stay Hydrated:**
   - Drink at least 8–10 glasses of water daily to support detoxification.
2. **Incorporate Detoxifying Herbs:**
   - **Dandelion root tea, milk thistle,** and **turmeric** can enhance liver function.
3. **Promote Regular Bowel Movements:**
   - Fiber-rich foods and probiotics help eliminate toxins and prevent reabsorption.

f. Support Thyroid Health
1. **Increase Selenium:**
   - **Sources**: Brazil nuts, seafood, and eggs.
   - **Benefits**: Protect the thyroid from oxidative stress.
2. **Boost Iodine:**
   - **Sources**: Seaweed, iodized salt.
   - **Benefits**: Essential for thyroid hormone production.
3. **Reduce Goitrogens:**
   - Avoid overconsumption of raw cruciferous vegetables if

you have thyroid issues.
g. Exercise for Hormonal Harmony
1. **Low-Impact Aerobics**:
   - Walking, swimming, or yoga can regulate cortisol levels and promote gut motility.
2. **Strength Training**:
   - Helps balance insulin and builds lean muscle, which supports hormonal health.
3. **Mind-Body Exercises**:
   - Pilates or tai chi can reduce stress while enhancing core strength.

h. Consider Supplementation
1. **Probiotics**:
   - Improve microbial diversity and support gut-hormone communication.
2. **Omega-3 Fatty Acids**:
   - Reduce inflammation and support hormone production.
3. **Adaptogens**:
   - Herbs like ashwagandha and rhodiola regulate cortisol and stress response.
4. **Magnesium**:
   - Promotes relaxation and reduces PMS symptoms.

4. Monitoring Hormonal Health and Wellness
a. Track Symptoms
- Keep a journal of symptoms such as bloating, mood swings, fatigue, or irregular cycles to identify patterns.

b. Regular Testing
- Consult your healthcare provider for tests that assess hormone levels, thyroid function, and gut health.

c. Adjust Lifestyle Practices
- Continuously tweak your diet, exercise, and stress management routines based on how your body responds.

5. Beyond Hormones: Fostering Overall Wellness
a. Foster Emotional Well-Being
- Build supportive relationships, engage in hobbies, and practice

gratitude.

b. Stay Active in Nature
- Regular exposure to sunlight boosts vitamin D levels, essential for hormonal balance and mood regulation.

c. Limit Environmental Toxins
- Reduce exposure to endocrine disruptors found in plastics, personal care products, and household cleaners.

Balancing Hormones Naturally: Using Food, Supplements, and Lifestyle Changes Post-Leaky Gut Healing

After healing leaky gut, the next step in your health journey is to address the intricate relationship between the gut and hormones. Hormones regulate everything from energy levels and mood to metabolism and reproductive health. A healthy gut provides the foundation for balanced hormones, but targeted strategies using **food**, **supplements**, and **lifestyle changes** are essential for long-term hormone health.

This chapter will guide you through practical, natural ways to balance hormones and maintain overall wellness after addressing leaky gut.

1. The Connection Between Gut Health and Hormones

Hormones are chemical messengers that influence numerous bodily functions. The gut plays a critical role in hormone regulation, affecting their production, metabolism, and detoxification.

How Gut Health Impacts Hormones:

1. **Microbiome Support:**
   - Gut bacteria produce and regulate key hormones such as serotonin (mood) and ghrelin (hunger).
   - The gut's **estrobolome** (a collection of bacteria) metabolizes estrogen. Dysbiosis in this area can lead to estrogen dominance, causing menstrual irregularities, mood swings, and bloating.
2. **Inflammation and Hormones:**
   - A healed gut reduces systemic inflammation, which helps regulate cortisol, thyroid hormones, and insulin.
3. **Nutrient Absorption:**
   - A healthy gut improves nutrient absorption, ensuring

essential vitamins and minerals for hormone synthesis are available.

2. Using Food to Balance Hormones

Food is one of the most powerful tools for naturally balancing hormones. A nutrient-dense, whole-food diet supports hormone production, detoxification, and stability.

a. Healthy Fats for Hormone Production

Hormones like estrogen, progesterone, and testosterone are made from cholesterol, so healthy fats are essential.

- **Sources**: Avocados, olive oil, coconut oil, nuts, seeds, fatty fish (salmon, mackerel, sardines).
- **Benefits**: Provide the building blocks for hormone synthesis and reduce inflammation.

b. Fiber for Detoxification

Fiber binds to excess hormones (like estrogen) in the gut, aiding in their elimination.

- **Sources**: Flaxseeds, chia seeds, leafy greens, broccoli, Brussels sprouts, whole grains.
- **Benefits**: Helps regulate estrogen levels and supports a healthy microbiome.

c. Cruciferous Vegetables for Estrogen Balance

Cruciferous vegetables contain **indole-3-carbinol**, which helps detoxify excess estrogen.

- **Sources**: Broccoli, cauliflower, kale, cabbage, arugula.
- **Benefits**: Supports liver detoxification and reduces the risk of estrogen dominance.

d. Protein for Hormonal Stability

Protein provides amino acids needed for hormone production and blood sugar stability.

- **Sources**: Organic chicken, grass-fed beef, eggs, lentils, quinoa.
- **Benefits**: Stabilizes insulin and cortisol levels, key hormones for energy and metabolism.

e. Anti-Inflammatory Foods

Reducing inflammation is key to hormonal balance.

- **Sources**: Turmeric, ginger, berries, leafy greens, walnuts.

- **Benefits**: Lowers cortisol and promotes thyroid health.

3. Supplements to Support Hormone Health

While food provides the foundation, supplements can fill gaps and offer additional support for hormone balance.

a. Magnesium
- **Role**: Reduces cortisol, supports progesterone production, and alleviates PMS symptoms.
- **Sources**: Magnesium glycinate or citrate.
- **Dosage**: 200–400 mg daily.

b. Omega-3 Fatty Acids
- **Role**: Reduce inflammation and support hormone production.
- **Sources**: Fish oil supplements.
- **Dosage**: 1–2 grams daily.

c. Vitamin D
- **Role**: Regulates insulin, thyroid, and reproductive hormones.
- **Sources**: Supplements or natural sunlight.
- **Dosage**: 2,000–4,000 IU daily (check with a healthcare provider).

d. Adaptogenic Herbs
- **Ashwagandha**: Balances cortisol and reduces stress.
- **Maca Root**: Boosts energy and regulates estrogen and progesterone.
- **Rhodiola Rosea**: Improves resilience to stress and stabilizes adrenal hormones.

e. Probiotics
- **Role**: Restore gut microbiome balance, which directly impacts estrogen metabolism and serotonin production.
- **Sources**: High-quality, multi-strain probiotic supplements.
- **Dosage**: 10–20 billion CFUs daily.

f. Zinc
- **Role**: Supports thyroid function and testosterone production.
- **Sources**: Zinc gluconate or zinc citrate.
- **Dosage**: 15–30 mg daily.

4. Lifestyle Changes for Hormonal Balance

Lifestyle habits play a pivotal role in supporting hormone health, working in tandem with diet and supplements.

a. Stress Management

Chronic stress disrupts cortisol levels, which can negatively impact other hormones.

- **Techniques**:
    - Mindfulness meditation: Practice 10–15 minutes daily to reduce stress.
    - Deep breathing: Try diaphragmatic breathing to activate the parasympathetic nervous system.
    - Yoga: Focus on poses like Child's Pose and Supine Twist to calm the nervous system.

b. Prioritize Sleep

Quality sleep regulates cortisol, insulin, and melatonin, ensuring overall hormonal balance.

- **Tips**:
    - Maintain a consistent sleep schedule.
    - Create a sleep-friendly environment with blackout curtains and cool temperatures.
    - Avoid screens 1–2 hours before bed to enhance melatonin production.

c. Exercise Regularly

Physical activity helps balance insulin, cortisol, and reproductive hormones.

- **Types**:
    - Strength training: Boosts testosterone and improves metabolism.
    - Low-impact cardio: Walking, swimming, or cycling supports cortisol regulation.
    - Yoga or Pilates: Enhances relaxation and strengthens the core.

d. Support Liver Detoxification

The liver metabolizes and detoxifies hormones like estrogen. Supporting liver health is crucial for hormonal balance.

- **Practices**:
    - Stay hydrated: Drink 8–10 glasses of water daily.
    - Eat liver-supportive foods: Garlic, beets, dandelion

greens, and turmeric.
- Reduce alcohol: Limit consumption to avoid overburdening the liver.

e. Maintain Balanced Blood Sugar

Fluctuations in blood sugar lead to insulin spikes, which disrupt cortisol and reproductive hormones.

- **Tips**:
  - Avoid refined sugars and carbs.
  - Eat smaller, balanced meals every 3–4 hours to maintain steady glucose levels.
  - Include protein and healthy fats in every meal.

5. Monitoring Progress and Staying Consistent

a. Track Symptoms

- Keep a journal to monitor symptoms like mood swings, energy levels, and menstrual changes.
- Note improvements in digestion, sleep, and stress levels.

b. Regular Testing

- Consult your healthcare provider for regular hormone level testing (e.g., estrogen, progesterone, cortisol, thyroid).

c. Adjust as Needed

- If symptoms persist, work with a practitioner to adjust your diet, supplements, or lifestyle changes.

6. Putting It All Together: A Day in the Life of Hormone Balance

Morning:
- Wake up with a glass of warm water and lemon for liver support.
- Breakfast: A smoothie with spinach, flaxseeds, avocado, and protein powder.
- Morning mindfulness: 10 minutes of meditation.

Midday:
- Lunch: Grilled salmon with roasted Brussels sprouts and quinoa.
- Take probiotics and omega-3 supplements.
- Post-meal walk to stabilize blood sugar.

Afternoon:
- Snack: Handful of almonds and a green tea.

- Practice deep breathing for 5 minutes to reduce stress.

Evening:
- Dinner: Chicken stir-fry with broccoli, ginger, and turmeric over cauliflower rice.
- Take magnesium and adaptogenic herbs like ashwagandha.
- Unwind with yoga or journaling before bed.

Gut and Mental Health: How Healing Your Gut Can Improve Mood, Mental Clarity, and Reduce Anxiety and Depression

The **gut-brain connection** is one of the most significant revelations in modern health science. Often referred to as the "second brain," the gut is intricately connected to our emotions, mental clarity, and overall psychological well-being. This relationship is mediated through the **gut-brain axis**, a two-way communication network that links the gut and brain through the **vagus nerve**, **immune system**, and **hormonal pathways**.

Healing your gut doesn't just improve digestion—it can profoundly affect your mood, mental clarity, and resilience against conditions like anxiety and depression. This chapter explores the gut-brain connection, the role of the microbiome, and actionable steps to support both gut and mental health.

1. Understanding the Gut-Brain Connection

The gut and brain are connected through several key mechanisms:

a. The Vagus Nerve
- The **vagus nerve** is the primary communication highway between the gut and brain. Signals from the gut microbiome can influence brain activity and vice versa.
- A healthy gut sends positive signals that promote calmness and clarity, while an imbalanced gut can signal stress, leading to anxiety and mood disorders.

b. The Microbiome and Neurotransmitters
- The gut microbiome produces **neurotransmitters** such as:
    - **Serotonin**: Often called the "happiness hormone," about **90% of serotonin** is produced in the gut.
    - **GABA**: A calming neurotransmitter that reduces anxiety.
    - **Dopamine**: Regulates motivation and pleasure.

- Imbalances in gut bacteria can impair the production of these neurotransmitters, directly affecting mood and mental clarity.

c. Inflammation and Mental Health
- A leaky gut or dysbiosis can trigger systemic inflammation, which is linked to anxiety, depression, and brain fog.
- Inflammation increases the production of stress hormones like **cortisol**, disrupting mental well-being.

d. Hormonal Pathways
- The gut regulates hormones like **cortisol** and **insulin**, which influence mood and energy levels.
- An unhealthy gut can lead to hormonal imbalances that exacerbate anxiety and depression.

2. How Gut Health Affects Mood and Mental Clarity

a. Anxiety
- Studies have shown that gut dysbiosis increases anxiety by disrupting GABA production and amplifying stress signals to the brain.

b. Depression
- An imbalanced gut microbiome reduces serotonin availability, contributing to feelings of sadness, low energy, and hopelessness.

c. Brain Fog
- Poor gut health impairs nutrient absorption (e.g., B vitamins, magnesium) critical for cognitive function, leading to brain fog and difficulty concentrating.

d. Stress Resilience
- A healthy gut improves stress resilience by regulating cortisol levels and reducing systemic inflammation.

3. Signs Your Gut May Be Affecting Your Mental Health
- Persistent feelings of anxiety or depression.
- Difficulty concentrating or frequent brain fog.
- Low energy or chronic fatigue.
- Worsening mood during digestive distress (e.g., bloating, diarrhea).
- Cravings for sugar or refined carbs, which can fuel harmful gut bacteria.

4. Healing the Gut to Improve Mental Health
a. Nourishing the Microbiome
The foundation of gut and mental health lies in a balanced and diverse microbiome.

- **Probiotic-Rich Foods**:
    - Include fermented foods like yogurt, kefir, sauerkraut, kimchi, and miso.
    - Benefits: Increase beneficial bacteria like *Lactobacillus* and *Bifidobacterium*, which are linked to reduced anxiety and depression.
- **Prebiotic-Rich Foods**:
    - Include foods like garlic, onions, asparagus, bananas, and oats to feed good bacteria.
    - Benefits: Enhance microbial diversity and support serotonin production.
- **Polyphenol-Rich Foods**:
    - Add dark chocolate, green tea, and berries, which promote beneficial gut bacteria.
    - Benefits: Reduce inflammation and support brain health.

b. Healing the Gut Lining
Repairing the gut lining reduces inflammation and improves mental clarity.

- **Bone Broth**:
    - High in collagen and amino acids like glutamine, which strengthen the gut barrier.
- **L-Glutamine**:
    - A supplement that repairs the intestinal lining and reduces leaky gut.
- **Zinc**:
    - Essential for gut repair and neurotransmitter production.

c. Reducing Inflammation
Lowering systemic inflammation is critical for better mental health.

- **Omega-3 Fatty Acids**:
    - Found in fatty fish (salmon, mackerel), chia seeds, and flaxseeds.

- Benefits: Reduce inflammation and improve mood.
- **Turmeric**:
  - Contains curcumin, a powerful anti-inflammatory compound.
  - Tip: Combine turmeric with black pepper to enhance absorption.

d. Managing Stress

Chronic stress disrupts the gut-brain axis, so stress management is crucial.

- **Mindfulness Meditation**:
  - Reduces cortisol and improves vagus nerve communication.
- **Breathing Exercises**:
  - Practice diaphragmatic breathing to calm the nervous system and improve digestion.
- **Yoga**:
  - Combines movement and breathwork to enhance gut-brain communication and reduce stress.

e. Optimizing Sleep

Sleep is essential for gut repair and neurotransmitter production.

- **Tips for Better Sleep**:
  - Maintain a consistent sleep schedule.
  - Avoid screens 1–2 hours before bed to promote melatonin production.
  - Drink chamomile tea or take magnesium before bed.

5. Supplements to Support Gut and Mental Health

a. Probiotics

- Look for multi-strain probiotics with *Lactobacillus* and *Bifidobacterium* species.
- Benefits: Improve serotonin production and reduce anxiety symptoms.

b. Omega-3 Fatty Acids

- Supplement if your diet lacks fatty fish.
- Benefits: Reduce inflammation and improve cognitive function.

c. Magnesium

- A calming mineral that regulates GABA production and reduces stress.
- Recommended dose: 200–400 mg of magnesium glycinate.

d. Vitamin D
- Regulates serotonin and supports a balanced microbiome.
- Dose: 2,000–4,000 IU daily (consult a healthcare provider).

e. Adaptogens
- **Ashwagandha**: Lowers cortisol and improves resilience to stress.
- **Rhodiola**: Boosts mood and mental clarity.

6. Lifestyle Changes for Long-Term Gut and Mental Health

a. Regular Physical Activity
- Exercise supports microbial diversity and reduces stress hormones.
- **Examples**: Walking, swimming, yoga, or strength training.

b. Limit Processed Foods
- Avoid refined sugars, artificial sweeteners, and processed carbs, which disrupt the microbiome and cause mood swings.

c. Connect with Nature
- Spending time in nature reduces stress and promotes mindfulness.
- Gardening or walking barefoot in the grass (grounding) can further support mental clarity.

d. Foster Social Connections
- Positive relationships and social interactions improve mood and reduce stress, indirectly benefiting the gut-brain axis.

7. Monitoring Progress

Tracking your gut and mental health can help you identify what works best for you.

- **Symptom Journal**:
  - Log daily mood, energy, and digestive symptoms.
- **Mindfulness Apps**:
  - Apps like Calm or Headspace can guide stress reduction techniques.
- **Regular Check-Ins**:

- Work with a healthcare provider to monitor improvements in mental health and gut function.

Maintaining a Healthy Gut Long-Term: Prevention and Maintenance for Optimal Gut Health

Healing your gut is a significant achievement, but long-term health requires consistent care and proactive prevention. A healthy gut is the foundation of overall wellness, influencing digestion, immunity, energy levels, mental health, and even hormonal balance. Once your gut is healed, adopting sustainable habits to maintain its health is essential for preventing issues like dysbiosis, leaky gut, and inflammation from recurring.

This chapter provides actionable strategies for keeping your gut in optimal shape through diet, lifestyle, and mindfulness practices.

1. The Importance of Long-Term Gut Maintenance

a. Why Maintenance Matters
- The gut is continuously exposed to factors like diet, stress, environmental toxins, and medications that can disrupt its balance.
- A healthy gut requires regular attention to maintain a thriving microbiome, strong intestinal lining, and low inflammation levels.

b. Benefits of a Healthy Gut
- Improved digestion and nutrient absorption.
- Enhanced immunity to fight infections and diseases.
- Better mood, mental clarity, and stress resilience through a balanced gut-brain axis.
- Regulation of hormones and blood sugar levels.

2. Dietary Habits for Long-Term Gut Health

a. Eat a Diverse Diet
- A varied diet promotes microbial diversity, a key marker of gut health.
- **Include:**
  - Vegetables: Spinach, kale, broccoli, carrots.
  - Fruits: Berries, apples, bananas.
  - Whole grains: Oats, quinoa, brown rice.

- Protein: Lean meats, fish, tofu, legumes.
- Healthy fats: Avocados, nuts, seeds, olive oil.

b. Focus on Prebiotic Foods
- Prebiotics are fibers that feed beneficial gut bacteria, ensuring their growth and activity.
- **Sources**: Garlic, onions, leeks, asparagus, bananas, chicory root, artichokes.

c. Incorporate Probiotic Foods Regularly
- Probiotic-rich foods replenish beneficial bacteria.
- **Examples**: Yogurt (with live cultures), kefir, sauerkraut, kimchi, miso, tempeh.

d. Limit Processed and Inflammatory Foods
- Avoid refined sugars, trans fats, artificial sweeteners (like aspartame), and processed foods, which disrupt the microbiome.
- Minimize gluten and dairy if they trigger symptoms for you.

e. Stay Hydrated
- Adequate water intake supports digestion, helps prevent constipation, and ensures proper mucosal lining in the gut.

f. Eat Mindfully
- Chew food thoroughly to ease digestion.
- Avoid overeating and practice mindful eating to reduce stress on the gut.

3. Lifestyle Practices for Gut Health

a. Manage Stress
- Chronic stress disrupts the gut-brain axis and harms the microbiome.
- **Techniques**:
  - **Meditation**: Spend 10–15 minutes daily practicing mindfulness.
  - **Yoga**: Gentle poses like Child's Pose and Cat-Cow can reduce stress and improve digestion.
  - **Deep Breathing**: Engage in diaphragmatic breathing to activate the parasympathetic nervous system.

b. Exercise Regularly
- Regular physical activity promotes microbial diversity and

supports healthy digestion.
- **Recommended Activities**:
    - Moderate cardio: Walking, cycling, swimming.
    - Strength training: Builds muscle and improves metabolic health.
    - Mind-body exercises: Yoga or Pilates to reduce stress and enhance core strength.

c. Prioritize Sleep
- Quality sleep is essential for gut repair and microbial balance.
- **Tips**:
    - Stick to a consistent sleep schedule.
    - Create a calming bedtime routine, free of screens and stimulants.
    - Consider magnesium or chamomile tea for better sleep.

d. Avoid Overuse of Medications
- Certain medications, like antibiotics, NSAIDs, and acid reducers, can harm the gut microbiome and lining.
- Use medications only when necessary and under guidance.
- Replenish probiotics after antibiotic use to restore microbial balance.

4. Environmental Factors and Gut Health

a. Reduce Exposure to Environmental Toxins
- Toxins like pesticides, plastics, and household chemicals can harm gut health.
- **Practical Tips**:
    - Choose organic produce when possible.
    - Avoid microwaving food in plastic containers.
    - Switch to non-toxic cleaning products.

b. Filter Your Water
- Use a water filter to remove chlorine, fluoride, and other chemicals that may disrupt the microbiome.

c. Spend Time Outdoors
- Regular exposure to nature increases microbial diversity and strengthens the immune system.
- Activities like gardening or hiking can introduce beneficial

microbes from the environment.

5. Regular Gut Health Checks
a. Pay Attention to Symptoms
- Monitor your body for signs of gut distress, such as bloating, constipation, diarrhea, or food sensitivities.
- Address symptoms promptly to prevent further issues.

b. Use a Food and Symptom Journal
- Track meals, symptoms, and stress levels to identify triggers or patterns.
- Adjust your diet and lifestyle based on what works for your gut.

c. Seek Professional Guidance
- Periodically consult a healthcare provider or nutritionist to ensure your gut health is on track.
- Consider gut microbiome testing for a detailed understanding of your gut bacteria composition.

6. Supplements for Gut Maintenance
a. Probiotics
- Regularly supplement with a high-quality, multi-strain probiotic to maintain microbial balance.
- Choose probiotics with strains like *Lactobacillus* and *Bifidobacterium*.

b. Prebiotics
- If dietary intake is insufficient, consider prebiotic supplements like inulin or fructooligosaccharides (FOS).

c. Digestive Enzymes
- Take digestive enzymes if you experience occasional bloating or difficulty digesting certain foods.

d. Omega-3 Fatty Acids
- Supplement with fish oil to reduce inflammation and support gut lining integrity.

e. L-Glutamine
- This amino acid helps maintain the gut lining and can be taken as needed for additional support.

7. Preventing Gut Imbalances
a. Rotate Your Diet

- Eating the same foods repeatedly can limit microbial diversity. Rotate your diet to introduce new nutrients and prevent sensitivities.

b. Avoid Overeating
- Overeating can strain digestion and disrupt the balance of gut bacteria.

c. Limit Alcohol and Caffeine
- Excessive alcohol and caffeine intake can irritate the gut lining and disrupt the microbiome.

8. Building Resilience Against Stressors

a. Strengthen the Vagus Nerve
- The vagus nerve connects the gut and brain, and strengthening it can improve resilience.
- **Practices**:
  - Deep breathing.
  - Singing or humming.
  - Cold exposure (e.g., a cold splash of water on the face).

b. Cultivate Social Connections
- Positive relationships and social interactions lower stress and support a healthier gut-brain axis.

c. Stay Consistent
- The key to long-term gut health is consistency. Small, daily habits compound into lasting benefits.

Chapter 9: Success Stories: Real Women Who Healed Their Gut

Hearing real-life success stories can be incredibly inspiring and motivating, especially when embarking on a health journey. In this chapter, we share the transformative stories of women who healed their guts, reclaimed their health, and improved their quality of life. These accounts not only highlight the challenges they faced but also showcase the strategies and habits that helped them succeed.

1. Sarah's Journey: Overcoming IBS and Chronic Fatigue
The Challenge

For years, Sarah, a 32-year-old teacher, struggled with **Irritable Bowel Syndrome (IBS)**. She experienced constant bloating, abdominal pain, and irregular bowel movements. The chronic fatigue that accompanied her symptoms made it difficult to get through the day, let alone enjoy her life.

Her Approach
- **Dietary Changes**:
    - Eliminated gluten, dairy, and processed foods.
    - Focused on an anti-inflammatory diet rich in vegetables, lean proteins, and healthy fats.
    - Incorporated fermented foods like kimchi and kefir for

probiotics.
- **Supplements**:
    - Took L-glutamine to repair her gut lining.
    - Used a multi-strain probiotic daily.
- **Lifestyle Adjustments**:
    - Practiced yoga three times a week to manage stress.
    - Began journaling to identify food triggers.

The Outcome

After six months of consistent effort, Sarah's symptoms improved dramatically. She now enjoys a regular digestive rhythm, no longer feels fatigued, and has the energy to pursue her passion for hiking. Sarah emphasizes the importance of staying patient and trusting the process.

2. Emily's Transformation: Healing from Leaky Gut and Autoimmune Symptoms

The Challenge

Emily, a 40-year-old graphic designer, was diagnosed with **Hashimoto's thyroiditis,** an autoimmune condition, after experiencing fatigue, brain fog, and weight gain. She discovered that leaky gut was exacerbating her symptoms.

Her Approach

- **Gut-Healing Diet**:
    - Adopted a Paleo-style diet, avoiding gluten, grains, dairy, and sugar.
    - Focused on bone broth, leafy greens, and wild-caught fish.
- **Stress Reduction**:
    - Implemented daily meditation and deep breathing exercises to reduce cortisol levels.
- **Targeted Supplements**:
    - Took zinc and selenium to support thyroid function.
    - Used digestive enzymes to improve nutrient absorption.

The Outcome

Within eight months, Emily noticed significant improvements in her energy levels and mental clarity. Her autoimmune symptoms are now well-managed, and she feels empowered to make informed choices about her health.

3. Rachel's Recovery: Beating Bloating and Food Intolerances

The Challenge

Rachel, a 27-year-old marketing professional, suffered from severe bloating, food intolerances, and occasional skin flare-ups. These issues began affecting her self-confidence and social life.

Her Approach
- **Food and Symptom Tracking**:
    - Kept a detailed food diary to identify triggers.
    - Found that gluten, dairy, and soy were causing her symptoms.
- **Microbiome Restoration**:
    - Focused on gut-friendly foods like asparagus, garlic, and bananas.
    - Introduced kombucha and sauerkraut for probiotics.
- **Exercise and Movement**:
    - Started Pilates to strengthen her core and improve digestion.

The Outcome

After following a gut-healing plan for five months, Rachel's bloating disappeared, and her food intolerances reduced significantly. She regained her confidence and learned how to maintain her gut health long-term.

4. Anna's Breakthrough: Conquering Anxiety and Digestive Issues

The Challenge

Anna, a 35-year-old mother of two, struggled with anxiety and frequent digestive discomfort, including constipation and heartburn. Her symptoms worsened during periods of stress, affecting her mood and family life.

Her Approach
- **Mindful Eating**:
    - Avoided eating on the go and practiced mindful eating techniques.
- **Stress Management**:

- Took up guided meditation and joined a weekly yoga class.
- **Gut Repair**:
    - Focused on healing her gut lining with L-glutamine and collagen supplements.
    - Drank herbal teas like chamomile and peppermint for digestion.

The Outcome

Over time, Anna noticed a significant reduction in her anxiety levels and digestive symptoms. Her newfound calmness allowed her to enjoy time with her children without constant worry.

5. Olivia's Victory: Addressing PCOS and Gut Health

The Challenge

Olivia, a 29-year-old chef, was diagnosed with **Polycystic Ovary Syndrome (PCOS)**. Her symptoms included hormonal imbalances, irregular periods, and persistent bloating.

Her Approach

- **Hormone-Friendly Diet**:
    - Focused on fiber-rich foods to eliminate excess estrogen.
    - Added cruciferous vegetables like broccoli and Brussels sprouts.
- **Supplement Support**:
    - Used probiotics to restore microbial balance.
    - Took magnesium and omega-3s to regulate hormones.
- **Regular Exercise**:
    - Combined strength training with low-impact cardio to stabilize blood sugar.

The Outcome

Within six months, Olivia's bloating subsided, her menstrual cycles became more regular, and her overall energy improved. She attributes her success to integrating gut health strategies with hormonal support.

Lessons Learned from Their Stories

1. Patience and Consistency Are Key

- Each woman's journey took several months of consistent effort before significant improvements were seen.

2. Tailored Approaches Work Best
- A one-size-fits-all approach doesn't work. Identifying triggers, whether dietary or lifestyle-related, was a critical part of their success.

3. Long-Term Commitment
- These women didn't just heal their gut—they committed to maintaining gut health as a long-term priority.

4. Mind-Body Connection Matters
- Stress management played a pivotal role in each success story, highlighting the importance of holistic healing.

Case Studies: Real-Life Success Stories of Women Who Healed Their Leaky Gut

Healing **leaky gut** is often a transformative journey that extends beyond digestive health. When the gut lining is restored, the body begins to function optimally, leading to improved hormonal balance, energy levels, and overall well-being. In this chapter, we highlight real-life success stories of women who have overcome leaky gut and experienced profound changes in their health. These case studies illustrate the power of holistic approaches and serve as inspiration for those embarking on their own healing journey.

Case Study 1: Emma's Story – Balancing Hormones and Boosting Energy

The Challenge

Emma, a 35-year-old accountant, experienced **irregular menstrual cycles**, low energy, and frequent mood swings. Despite eating a relatively healthy diet, she felt fatigued and struggled with weight gain around her midsection. A visit to a functional medicine practitioner revealed **leaky gut syndrome** and **hormonal imbalances**, including estrogen dominance.

Her Approach

1. **Dietary Changes**:
   - Emma eliminated gluten, dairy, and refined sugar from her diet.
   - She introduced gut-healing foods such as bone broth, leafy greens, and healthy fats like avocado and olive oil.

- She incorporated cruciferous vegetables (broccoli, kale, cauliflower) to support estrogen detoxification.
2. **Supplements**:
   - Took a high-quality probiotic with strains like *Lactobacillus* and *Bifidobacterium* to restore her gut microbiome.
   - Used L-glutamine and collagen to repair her intestinal lining.
   - Added magnesium and zinc to support hormone regulation.
3. **Lifestyle Adjustments**:
   - Practiced mindfulness meditation for 10 minutes daily to reduce stress.
   - Started yoga twice a week to improve circulation and lower cortisol levels.

The Results

After six months of following her protocol, Emma noticed significant improvements. Her menstrual cycle normalized, her energy levels skyrocketed, and her mood swings diminished. She also shed excess weight, particularly around her abdomen, and feels empowered to maintain her health.

Case Study 2: Mia's Journey – Conquering Fatigue and Improving Mental Clarity

The Challenge

Mia, a 29-year-old nurse, struggled with **chronic fatigue**, frequent bloating, and brain fog. She often felt overwhelmed at work and had difficulty concentrating. After extensive research, Mia suspected **leaky gut syndrome** was the root cause of her issues.

Her Approach

1. **Gut-Healing Diet**:
   - Mia transitioned to an anti-inflammatory diet, cutting out processed foods, alcohol, and caffeine.
   - She focused on prebiotic foods like garlic, asparagus, and bananas, along with fermented foods like sauerkraut and kefir.

- She avoided known triggers such as gluten and soy.
2. **Supplements**:
    - Took digestive enzymes to enhance nutrient absorption.
    - Supplemented with omega-3 fatty acids to reduce inflammation.
    - Used adaptogens like ashwagandha to regulate stress responses.
3. **Stress Management**:
    - Implemented deep breathing exercises during her work breaks.
    - Scheduled daily 20-minute walks outdoors to calm her mind and promote gut-brain axis health.

The Results
Within four months, Mia's brain fog lifted, and her energy levels improved dramatically. She now manages her busy workdays with greater ease and no longer feels bloated after meals. Mia's success has motivated her to continue prioritizing her gut health.

Case Study 3: Olivia's Success – Healing PCOS and Leaky Gut
The Challenge
Olivia, a 32-year-old teacher, was diagnosed with **Polycystic Ovary Syndrome (PCOS)** and **leaky gut syndrome** after experiencing irregular periods, weight gain, and acne. Her gut issues were exacerbating her hormonal imbalance, leading to worsening PCOS symptoms.

Her Approach
1. **Customized Nutrition Plan**:
    - Focused on an anti-inflammatory diet rich in fiber to stabilize blood sugar and support hormone regulation.
    - Added flaxseeds, chia seeds, and leafy greens to support estrogen metabolism.
    - Avoided inflammatory foods like dairy, processed oils, and refined carbs.
2. **Gut Repair Protocol**:
    - Drank bone broth daily to strengthen her gut lining.
    - Took a prebiotic and probiotic combination to diversify her gut microbiome.

- Supplemented with L-glutamine and vitamin D.
3. **Lifestyle Changes**:
    - Implemented strength training and yoga to stabilize her insulin levels and reduce cortisol.
    - Practiced gratitude journaling to shift her mindset and reduce stress.

The Results

After five months, Olivia noticed significant improvements. Her menstrual cycle became regular, her acne cleared, and she lost weight without restrictive dieting. She credits her success to healing her gut, which had a ripple effect on her hormonal health.

Case Study 4: Sophia's Breakthrough – Reversing Autoimmune Symptoms

The Challenge

Sophia, a 40-year-old lawyer, was diagnosed with **Hashimoto's thyroiditis**, an autoimmune thyroid disorder. She experienced fatigue, joint pain, and weight gain, along with digestive issues like bloating and constipation. Testing revealed **leaky gut syndrome** as a contributing factor to her autoimmune condition.

Her Approach

1. **Elimination Diet**:
    - Sophia removed gluten, dairy, and nightshades (e.g., tomatoes, peppers) to reduce inflammation.
    - She focused on nutrient-dense foods like wild-caught salmon, sweet potatoes, and dark leafy greens.
    - She included anti-inflammatory spices like turmeric and ginger in her meals.
2. **Supplements**:
    - Took selenium and zinc to support thyroid function.
    - Used probiotics to restore microbial diversity.
    - Supplemented with glutathione to reduce oxidative stress.
3. **Stress and Sleep Management**:
    - Started a nightly wind-down routine, including chamomile tea and guided meditation.

- Focused on improving sleep hygiene by keeping her bedroom dark and electronics-free.

The Results

Within six months, Sophia felt like a new person. Her energy levels rebounded, her digestive issues resolved, and her thyroid function improved significantly. Her autoimmune symptoms are now well-managed, and she enjoys a more active lifestyle.

Case Study 5: Rachel's Renewal – Addressing Anxiety and Digestive Issues

The Challenge

Rachel, a 28-year-old entrepreneur, suffered from **anxiety**, **frequent diarrhea**, and abdominal pain. These issues disrupted her productivity and personal life. After visiting a nutritionist, Rachel learned that **leaky gut syndrome** and stress were fueling her symptoms.

Her Approach

1. **Healing Foods**:
   - Switched to a Mediterranean diet rich in whole foods, healthy fats, and lean proteins.
   - Drank peppermint tea to soothe her digestive system.
   - Added fermented foods like yogurt and kombucha to her daily routine.
2. **Supplements**:
   - Took magnesium to calm her nervous system and regulate bowel movements.
   - Used a high-quality probiotic to rebuild her microbiome.
   - Supplemented with collagen to repair her gut lining.
3. **Stress Reduction**:
   - Joined a local yoga studio and attended classes twice a week.
   - Practiced mindfulness meditation for 15 minutes every morning.

The Results

After four months, Rachel's anxiety decreased significantly, and her digestion improved. She feels more grounded and productive, crediting her success to a combination of gut healing and stress management.

Lessons Learned
1. **Gut Healing Is Holistic**:
   - Addressing diet, stress, and lifestyle simultaneously led to the best outcomes.
2. **Patience Pays Off**:
   - Results took time, but consistency and persistence were critical.
3. **Individualized Approaches Work**:
   - Each woman tailored her protocol to fit her unique symptoms and goals.

Before-and-After Transformations: Inspiring Stories of Personal Health Journeys

Transforming health can often feel like an overwhelming and daunting process, especially for those struggling with chronic issues like gut problems, hormonal imbalances, and fatigue. However, countless individuals have experienced remarkable "before-and-after" transformations that showcase the power of commitment, education, and lifestyle changes. These stories offer hope and reassurance that healing is possible, even in the face of long-standing health challenges.

In this chapter, we highlight inspiring personal journeys that demonstrate the profound physical, mental, and emotional shifts that can occur when individuals take charge of their health. These stories remind readers that, with patience and persistence, they too can achieve similar results.

Transformation 1: Jessica's Journey – From Gut Struggles to Vibrant Energy

Before: Constant Bloating and Exhaustion

Jessica, a 34-year-old marketing executive, dealt with **chronic bloating**, irregular bowel movements, and extreme fatigue. Her symptoms worsened after stressful deadlines, leaving her irritable and drained. Visits to multiple doctors yielded no clear answers, leaving her feeling defeated.

The Turning Point

Jessica began researching gut health and learned about **leaky gut syndrome**. After seeking guidance from a functional nutritionist, she decided to commit to a gut-healing program.

After: Renewed Energy and Confidence

Six months later, Jessica experienced a complete transformation. Her bloating disappeared, her energy levels soared, and she regained confidence in her ability to handle work and social commitments. Jessica credits her transformation to:

- Switching to an anti-inflammatory diet, rich in vegetables, lean proteins, and fermented foods.
- Regular yoga practice to manage stress.
- A daily probiotic supplement and L-glutamine to heal her gut lining.

Jessica now inspires others by sharing her story and empowering them to prioritize their health.

Transformation 2: Maria's Triumph – From Hormonal Imbalances to Harmony

Before: Struggling with PCOS Symptoms

Maria, a 28-year-old teacher, was diagnosed with **Polycystic Ovary Syndrome (PCOS)** after experiencing irregular periods, severe acne, and unexplainable weight gain. Despite following various diets, her symptoms persisted, leaving her frustrated and hopeless.

The Turning Point

Maria discovered the link between gut health and hormonal balance. With this knowledge, she shifted her focus from calorie restriction to **healing her gut**.

After: Balanced Hormones and Clear Skin

Within eight months, Maria experienced life-changing results:

- Her menstrual cycle became regular for the first time in years.
- Her acne cleared, and her skin glowed with health.
- She lost 15 pounds naturally, without extreme dieting.

Maria's transformation involved:

- Adopting a high-fiber diet with prebiotic foods like flaxseeds and leafy greens.
- Eliminating sugar and processed foods that were inflaming her gut.
- Using supplements like magnesium and probiotics to support

hormone regulation.

Maria now feels empowered and shares her journey with others navigating similar struggles.

Transformation 3: Hannah's Success – From Anxiety and Brain Fog to Mental Clarity

Before: Overwhelmed by Anxiety

Hannah, a 32-year-old graphic designer, struggled with **anxiety**, **brain fog**, and poor digestion. Her symptoms often interfered with her creative work, leaving her feeling defeated and uninspired.

The Turning Point

Hannah read about the **gut-brain connection** and realized her anxiety might be tied to her gut health. She decided to embark on a journey to heal her gut and manage her stress.

After: A Clear Mind and Calm Spirit

Four months into her transformation, Hannah felt like a new person:
- Her anxiety diminished significantly, and she felt more emotionally balanced.
- She regained mental clarity, boosting her creativity and productivity at work.
- Her digestion improved, eliminating the discomfort she once felt daily.

Hannah's transformation included:
- Practicing daily mindfulness meditation to reduce stress.
- Incorporating probiotic-rich foods like kefir and sauerkraut into her meals.
- Drinking herbal teas like chamomile and peppermint to soothe her gut.

Today, Hannah advocates for mental health and gut healing as interconnected pathways to wellness.

Transformation 4: Lisa's Turnaround – From Chronic Fatigue to Thriving Health

Before: Drained and Dependent on Caffeine

Lisa, a 40-year-old mother of three, relied on coffee to get through her day. She struggled with **chronic fatigue**, **irritability**, and frequent sugar cravings. Despite trying various diets and exercise routines, her energy levels remained low, and she felt stuck in a cycle of exhaustion.

The Turning Point

A friend recommended Lisa look into **gut healing** as a potential solution. Skeptical but desperate, Lisa decided to try it.

After: Vibrant Energy and Newfound Vitality

Six months later, Lisa was amazed by her transformation:
- She no longer needed caffeine to wake up or sugar to keep her going.
- She felt energized, positive, and capable of handling her busy life.
- Her sugar cravings vanished, and she developed a healthier relationship with food.

Lisa attributes her transformation to:
- Following a whole-food diet with plenty of healthy fats, like avocado and salmon.
- Taking a daily probiotic and omega-3 supplement to reduce inflammation.
- Prioritizing sleep and creating a nighttime wind-down routine.

Lisa now enjoys her days with her children and shares her story to inspire other moms to prioritize their health.

Transformation 5: Emily's Recovery – From Autoimmune Symptoms to Wellness

Before: Battling Hashimoto's Thyroiditis

Emily, a 36-year-old nurse, faced debilitating symptoms from **Hashimoto's thyroiditis**, including joint pain, brain fog, and weight gain. Her condition left her feeling defeated and uncertain about her future.

The Turning Point

After learning about the role of gut health in autoimmune conditions, Emily sought help from a holistic practitioner who created a personalized gut-healing plan.

After: Symptom-Free Living

Eight months later, Emily's life took a dramatic turn:
- Her joint pain disappeared, and she felt stronger and more mobile.
- Her brain fog lifted, allowing her to excel in her nursing career.

- She achieved a healthy weight and improved her thyroid function.

Emily's transformation involved:
- Eliminating gluten and dairy from her diet to reduce inflammation.
- Drinking bone broth and taking L-glutamine to repair her gut lining.
- Incorporating mindfulness practices to lower stress and support her immune system.

Emily is now symptom-free and encourages others with autoimmune conditions to explore gut healing.

Lessons from Their Transformations
1. **Patience is Key**:
   - None of these women achieved their results overnight. Their transformations required time, consistency, and dedication.
2. **Holistic Approaches Work**:
   - Addressing diet, lifestyle, and stress simultaneously proved essential for sustainable change.
3. **Individualized Plans Are Crucial**:
   - Each journey was unique, highlighting the importance of tailoring strategies to individual needs and symptoms.
4. **Hope Is Real**:
   - These stories show that even when health issues feel overwhelming, transformation is possible.

Chapter 10: Frequently Asked Questions About Leaky Gut and Women's Health

Healing **leaky gut** can be a complex journey, especially as it often overlaps with broader health concerns such as hormonal imbalances, mental health, and autoimmune conditions. This chapter addresses some of the most common questions about leaky gut and its connection to women's health, providing clear and actionable insights to help readers understand and navigate their healing journey.

1. What Exactly Is Leaky Gut?

Leaky gut, also known as **increased intestinal permeability**, occurs when the lining of the small intestine becomes damaged. This damage allows toxins, undigested food particles, and harmful bacteria to "leak" into the bloodstream, triggering inflammation and immune responses.

Key Symptoms:
- Bloating, gas, and irregular bowel movements.
- Food sensitivities or intolerances.
- Fatigue, brain fog, and skin issues.
- Hormonal imbalances and mood changes.

Why It Matters for Women:

Leaky gut is often linked to hormonal disorders like **PCOS**, **endometriosis**, and **thyroid dysfunction**, making it especially important for women to address.

2. How Does Leaky Gut Affect Women's Hormonal Health?

The gut and hormones are deeply connected. A compromised gut can:

- **Disrupt Estrogen Metabolism**: A healthy gut microbiome helps detoxify estrogen. Dysbiosis (an imbalance of gut bacteria) can lead to estrogen dominance, causing bloating, mood swings, and irregular periods.
- **Elevate Cortisol Levels**: Leaky gut often triggers chronic stress, which increases cortisol and disrupts other hormones.
- **Impact Thyroid Health**: Leaky gut contributes to systemic inflammation, a key factor in autoimmune thyroid disorders like Hashimoto's.

3. What Causes Leaky Gut?

Several factors contribute to the development of leaky gut:

- **Dietary Triggers**:
    - Gluten, dairy, sugar, and processed foods are common culprits.
- **Chronic Stress**:
    - Prolonged stress weakens the gut lining and alters microbial balance.
- **Medications**:
    - Overuse of antibiotics, NSAIDs (e.g., ibuprofen), and antacids can damage the gut lining.
- **Toxins**:
    - Pesticides, heavy metals, and endocrine disruptors can harm the microbiome.
- **Underlying Conditions**:
    - Autoimmune disorders, infections, and small intestinal bacterial overgrowth (SIBO) often co-occur with leaky gut.

4. Can Healing Leaky Gut Improve Mental Health?

Yes, healing your gut can significantly improve mental health. The **gut-brain axis** is a two-way communication system that directly links gut health to mood and cognitive function.

How It Helps:
- Restoring the gut microbiome boosts the production of **serotonin** and **GABA**, neurotransmitters that regulate mood and anxiety.
- Reducing gut inflammation can lower systemic inflammation, which is linked to depression and brain fog.

5. What Are the Best Foods for Healing Leaky Gut?

Healing leaky gut requires an **anti-inflammatory, nutrient-rich diet** that supports the gut lining and microbiome.

Gut-Healing Foods:
- **Bone Broth**: High in collagen and amino acids like glutamine, which repair the gut lining.
- **Fermented Foods**: Yogurt, kefir, sauerkraut, and kimchi provide probiotics.
- **Prebiotic Foods**: Garlic, onions, asparagus, and bananas feed beneficial bacteria.
- **Leafy Greens and Vegetables**: Spinach, kale, broccoli, and carrots reduce inflammation.
- **Healthy Fats**: Avocado, olive oil, and coconut oil support gut health.

6. Are Supplements Necessary for Healing Leaky Gut?

While a nutrient-dense diet is the foundation, supplements can accelerate healing:
- **Probiotics**: Replenish beneficial bacteria and restore microbial balance.
- **L-Glutamine**: Repairs and strengthens the intestinal lining.
- **Digestive Enzymes**: Aid in breaking down food, reducing stress on the gut.
- **Omega-3 Fatty Acids**: Reduce inflammation and support the gut lining.
- **Vitamin D**: Regulates immune function and promotes a healthy microbiome.

7. Can I Exercise While Healing My Gut?

Yes, but moderation is key. Overexercising can elevate cortisol levels, worsening gut health.

Recommended Exercises:
- **Low-Impact Aerobics**: Walking, cycling, swimming.
- **Yoga or Pilates**: Focus on gentle movements and core strength.
- **Strength Training**: Promotes metabolic health and insulin sensitivity.

8. How Long Does It Take to Heal Leaky Gut?

Healing leaky gut is a gradual process that depends on the severity of the condition and the consistency of your efforts.

General Timeline:
- **Initial Improvements**: 4–6 weeks with a strict gut-healing protocol.
- **Significant Healing**: 3–6 months for most people.
- **Long-Term Maintenance**: Continuous care to prevent recurrence.

9. Can Leaky Gut Come Back After Healing?

Yes, if the underlying causes are not addressed. Preventative measures are crucial for long-term gut health.

Maintenance Tips:
- Stick to an anti-inflammatory diet.
- Manage stress through mindfulness practices.
- Avoid overuse of medications that harm the gut.
- Incorporate probiotics and prebiotics regularly.

10. Is Leaky Gut Linked to Autoimmune Disorders?

Yes, leaky gut is strongly associated with autoimmune conditions like:
- **Hashimoto's Thyroiditis**
- **Rheumatoid Arthritis**
- **Celiac Disease**
- **Lupus**

Why?

A leaky gut allows foreign particles to enter the bloodstream, triggering an immune response. Over time, this can lead to the development or worsening of autoimmune diseases.

11. Can Hormonal Birth Control Affect Gut Health?

Yes, hormonal birth control can disrupt gut health by:

- Altering microbial balance.
- Contributing to inflammation.
- Increasing the risk of leaky gut when combined with other stressors.

12. What Role Does Sleep Play in Gut Healing?
Sleep is critical for gut repair and overall health. Poor sleep disrupts the gut microbiome and weakens the intestinal barrier.

Tips for Better Sleep:
- Maintain a consistent sleep schedule.
- Avoid caffeine and screens before bed.
- Practice relaxation techniques like deep breathing or meditation.

13. Can Stress Alone Cause Leaky Gut?
Chronic stress is a significant contributor to leaky gut. It increases cortisol levels, which:
- Weakens the gut lining.
- Disrupts the balance of gut bacteria.
- Slows digestion, leading to further gut stress.

14. Are There Tests for Leaky Gut?
Yes, diagnostic tests can help identify leaky gut:
- **Zonulin Testing**: Measures levels of zonulin, a protein that regulates gut permeability.
- **Lactulose-Mannitol Test**: Assesses intestinal permeability by measuring sugar absorption.
- **Stool Analysis**: Evaluates gut bacteria, inflammation markers, and digestive function.

Consult a healthcare provider for testing recommendations.

15. How Do I Know If My Gut Is Healed?
Signs your gut is healing include:
- Improved digestion (less bloating, regular bowel movements).
- Reduced food sensitivities.
- Increased energy levels.
- Clearer skin and reduced inflammation.
- Better mood and mental clarity.

Addressing Common Myths: Dispelling Misconceptions About Leaky Gut

Leaky gut, or **increased intestinal permeability**, has gained significant attention in recent years, both in mainstream and alternative health circles. However, with this rising awareness comes a host of **myths and misconceptions** that can misinform individuals and prevent them from seeking effective solutions. In this chapter, we'll separate fact from fiction, dispel common myths, and provide evidence-based insights into the condition and its impact on overall health.

Myth 1: "Leaky gut is just a digestive problem."

The Truth: Leaky gut affects the entire body, not just digestion.

While digestive symptoms such as bloating, diarrhea, and food sensitivities are common indicators of leaky gut, the condition extends far beyond the gastrointestinal system.

- **Systemic Inflammation**: When the gut lining is compromised, harmful particles (e.g., toxins, undigested food, and bacteria) enter the bloodstream, triggering widespread inflammation. This can exacerbate conditions like arthritis, skin issues, and autoimmune diseases.
- **Mental Health**: The gut-brain connection means leaky gut can contribute to anxiety, depression, and brain fog by disrupting neurotransmitter production.
- **Hormonal Imbalances**: A leaky gut affects hormone regulation by interfering with nutrient absorption and increasing cortisol levels due to chronic inflammation.

Leaky gut is a systemic issue with far-reaching consequences, making it much more than just a digestive concern.

Myth 2: "Leaky gut isn't a real condition—there's no proven science."

The Truth: Leaky gut is supported by scientific evidence.

Although "leaky gut" is not an official medical diagnosis in traditional medicine, the concept of **increased intestinal permeability** is well-documented in scientific literature.

- **Zonulin**: Research shows that the protein **zonulin** regulates intestinal permeability. Elevated zonulin levels are linked to leaky gut and conditions like celiac disease and type 1 diabetes.
- **Autoimmune Diseases**: Studies have found a strong correlation

between leaky gut and autoimmune disorders such as Hashimoto's thyroiditis, rheumatoid arthritis, and lupus.
- **Gut Microbiome Research**: Disruption in the gut microbiome, a hallmark of leaky gut, has been extensively studied and linked to various health conditions, including IBS, obesity, and mental health disorders.

Leaky gut is not a fringe theory—it's a physiological phenomenon recognized in the scientific community, even if it is not universally accepted as a standalone diagnosis.

Myth 3: "Only people with digestive diseases get leaky gut."
The Truth: Anyone can develop leaky gut.

Leaky gut is not exclusive to individuals with pre-existing digestive disorders like IBS, Crohn's disease, or celiac disease. Several factors can compromise gut integrity in otherwise healthy individuals, including:
- **Diet**: A diet high in processed foods, sugar, and alcohol can damage the gut lining.
- **Stress**: Chronic stress elevates cortisol levels, which weakens the gut barrier.
- **Medications**: Overuse of antibiotics, NSAIDs, and antacids disrupts gut bacteria and damages the intestinal lining.
- **Environmental Toxins**: Exposure to pesticides, heavy metals, and pollutants can increase gut permeability.

Leaky gut can develop in anyone exposed to these triggers, making prevention and awareness essential for all.

Myth 4: "If I don't have symptoms, I don't have leaky gut."
The Truth: Leaky gut can exist without obvious symptoms.

Many individuals with leaky gut may not experience noticeable digestive issues but could exhibit symptoms in other areas of their health:
- **Skin**: Conditions like eczema, rosacea, and acne are often linked to gut permeability.
- **Mood and Cognition**: Brain fog, anxiety, and depression can result from disruptions in the gut-brain axis.
- **Immune System**: Frequent colds, allergies, or autoimmune flares may be signs of leaky gut.
- **Fatigue**: Chronic fatigue can stem from inflammation caused by

a compromised gut.

The absence of classic digestive symptoms does not rule out leaky gut. It's important to consider the condition's broader impacts on overall health.

Myth 5: "Leaky gut can be fixed with a single supplement."
The Truth: Healing leaky gut requires a holistic approach.

While certain supplements (e.g., probiotics, L-glutamine, and digestive enzymes) can play a vital role in repairing the gut, no single pill can address the multifaceted nature of leaky gut.

A comprehensive approach includes:
1. **Diet**: Focus on anti-inflammatory, nutrient-dense foods like bone broth, fermented foods, and prebiotic vegetables while avoiding processed foods, gluten, and dairy.
2. **Lifestyle**: Manage stress through mindfulness, yoga, and adequate sleep.
3. **Supplementation**: Use targeted supplements to repair the gut lining, restore microbial balance, and reduce inflammation.

Healing leaky gut is a process that requires consistency, dietary changes, and lifestyle adjustments, not just a quick fix.

Myth 6: "Leaky gut can be permanently cured."
The Truth: Gut health requires ongoing maintenance.

While leaky gut can be healed, the gut lining is constantly influenced by diet, lifestyle, and environmental factors. Without continued care, the condition can return.

- **Preventive Measures**:
    - Stick to an anti-inflammatory diet.
    - Manage stress and practice mindfulness.
    - Avoid overuse of medications that harm the gut lining (e.g., NSAIDs, antibiotics).

Gut health is dynamic, and maintaining a healthy gut requires lifelong attention and care.

Myth 7: "Leaky gut affects only adults."
The Truth: Leaky gut can affect individuals of all ages.

Children, teens, and older adults are all susceptible to leaky gut due to unique life stages and challenges:

- **Children**: Food sensitivities, environmental toxins, and high-sugar diets can contribute to gut permeability in kids.
- **Teens**: Stress from academics and hormonal changes can disrupt gut health.
- **Older Adults**: Aging naturally weakens the gut lining and microbiome diversity, increasing the risk of leaky gut.

Leaky gut is a condition that requires attention at all stages of life, not just adulthood.

Myth 8: "Leaky gut is a rare condition."
The Truth: Leaky gut is likely more common than we think.

Modern lifestyles filled with processed foods, chronic stress, and environmental toxins make leaky gut a widespread issue. While it may not always lead to noticeable symptoms, its effects can manifest in various forms, including inflammation, fatigue, and skin issues.

Raising awareness about leaky gut can help more people address its root causes and improve their overall health.

Myth 9: "I can't afford to heal my leaky gut."
The Truth: Gut healing can be budget-friendly.

While high-end supplements and specialty foods can help, there are plenty of affordable strategies to heal leaky gut:
- Focus on whole foods like vegetables, fruits, and legumes.
- Use natural, inexpensive remedies like bone broth and fermented vegetables.
- Prioritize stress management techniques like deep breathing and mindfulness, which are free and highly effective.

Healing leaky gut doesn't have to break the bank—it's about making sustainable, informed choices.

Myth 10: "Once I start healing, I'll see immediate results."
The Truth: Gut healing takes time and consistency.

The process of healing leaky gut varies depending on the individual and the severity of the condition. Most people begin to see improvements in **4–6 weeks**, but significant healing can take **3–6 months** or longer.

Consistency is key, and gradual progress should be celebrated. Patience and commitment lead to long-term success.

Answering Reader Questions: Healing Leaky Gut and Maintaining a Healthy Gut for Life

As you embark on the journey to heal leaky gut and maintain long-term gut health, questions often arise about the process, potential obstacles, and best practices. This chapter compiles and answers some of the most frequently asked questions, offering actionable advice and practical insights to help you navigate your path to a healthier gut and overall wellness.

1. How do I know if I have leaky gut?

Leaky gut can manifest in many ways, not all of which are limited to the digestive system. Common signs include:

- **Digestive symptoms**: Bloating, gas, diarrhea, constipation, or food sensitivities.
- **Skin issues**: Eczema, acne, or rosacea.
- **Mental health concerns**: Brain fog, anxiety, or depression.
- **Autoimmune disorders**: Hashimoto's thyroiditis, rheumatoid arthritis, or lupus.
- **Fatigue and low energy**: Often stemming from poor nutrient absorption.

If you suspect leaky gut, consult a healthcare professional. Tests like the **zonulin test** or the **lactulose-mannitol test** can help confirm intestinal permeability.

2. What's the best diet for healing leaky gut?

A gut-healing diet focuses on reducing inflammation, repairing the gut lining, and restoring microbial balance. Key principles include:

Foods to Include:

- **Gut-healing foods**: Bone broth, collagen, and L-glutamine-rich foods.
- **Prebiotic foods**: Garlic, onions, asparagus, and bananas.
- **Probiotic foods**: Yogurt, kefir, sauerkraut, and kimchi.
- **Anti-inflammatory foods**: Leafy greens, berries, and fatty fish like salmon.
- **Healthy fats**: Avocado, olive oil, and coconut oil.

Foods to Avoid:

- Gluten, dairy, and soy (common triggers).

- Refined sugar and artificial sweeteners.
- Processed and fried foods.
- Alcohol and excessive caffeine.

3. How long does it take to heal leaky gut?

The healing timeline varies depending on the severity of your condition and how consistently you follow a gut-healing plan.

- **Mild Cases**: Improvements may be seen in as little as 4–6 weeks.
- **Moderate to Severe Cases**: Healing can take 3–6 months or longer.

Consistency with diet, supplements, and lifestyle changes is crucial for sustained results.

4. What supplements help heal leaky gut?

Supplements can accelerate gut healing by addressing specific deficiencies and promoting repair.

Key Supplements:
1. **Probiotics**: Restore microbial balance.
    - Look for multi-strain probiotics with *Lactobacillus* and *Bifidobacterium*.
2. **L-Glutamine**: Repairs the gut lining.
    - Dosage: 5–10 grams daily.
3. **Collagen or Bone Broth Powder**: Strengthens the intestinal barrier.
4. **Digestive Enzymes**: Improve nutrient absorption and reduce digestive stress.
5. **Omega-3 Fatty Acids**: Reduce inflammation.
    - Dosage: 1–2 grams daily.
6. **Zinc**: Supports gut lining repair and immune health.
    - Dosage: 15–30 mg daily.
7. **Vitamin D**: Regulates immunity and microbial balance.
    - Dosage: 2,000–4,000 IU daily (check with your doctor).

5. Can I exercise while healing my gut?

Yes, but avoid overexertion, as intense exercise can increase cortisol levels and worsen gut permeability.

Best Exercises for Gut Healing:
- Low-impact activities: Walking, swimming, cycling.

- Yoga: Gentle poses like Child's Pose and Supine Twist to promote digestion.
- Strength training: Light resistance exercises to boost metabolism.

Aim for 30 minutes of moderate activity 3–5 times a week to support gut health without adding stress.

6. How does stress affect gut health, and how can I manage it?

Stress directly impacts the gut-brain axis, increasing cortisol levels and disrupting the gut microbiome. Chronic stress can worsen gut permeability and delay healing.

Stress Management Techniques:
- **Mindfulness meditation**: Spend 10–15 minutes daily focusing on your breath.
- **Deep breathing**: Practice diaphragmatic breathing to activate the parasympathetic nervous system.
- **Yoga or Tai Chi**: Combines movement and relaxation for stress relief.
- **Gratitude journaling**: Reflect on positive moments daily to reduce anxiety.

Stress management is as important as diet when it comes to healing your gut.

7. Can I drink alcohol while healing my gut?

Alcohol can irritate the gut lining, disrupt the microbiome, and delay healing. It's best to avoid alcohol entirely during the initial healing phase. If you reintroduce alcohol later, opt for **low-sugar options** like dry wine or spirits, and consume it sparingly.

8. What role does sleep play in gut healing?

Sleep is critical for gut repair and overall health. Poor sleep disrupts microbial diversity and weakens the gut barrier.

Tips for Better Sleep:
- Stick to a consistent sleep schedule.
- Avoid screens and stimulants (caffeine, alcohol) 1–2 hours before bedtime.
- Create a relaxing bedtime routine, such as drinking chamomile tea or reading.

9. How do I maintain gut health after it's healed?

Gut health is an ongoing commitment that requires sustainable habits.

Long-Term Maintenance Tips:
1. **Balanced Diet**: Continue eating a variety of whole, nutrient-dense foods.
2. **Probiotic and Prebiotic Foods**: Regularly include fermented foods and fiber-rich vegetables.
3. **Stay Hydrated**: Drink plenty of water to support digestion.
4. **Minimize Stress**: Incorporate mindfulness practices into your daily routine.
5. **Limit Harmful Medications**: Avoid overuse of NSAIDs, antibiotics, and antacids unless prescribed.
6. **Exercise Regularly**: Stay active with low to moderate-intensity workouts.

10. Can leaky gut come back after healing?

Yes, leaky gut can return if underlying triggers are not managed. Common causes of recurrence include:
- Reintroducing inflammatory foods.
- Chronic stress and lack of sleep.
- Environmental toxins or overuse of medications.

Adopting preventive measures like a balanced diet, stress management, and regular exercise can help keep your gut healthy for life.

11. Are food sensitivities permanent with leaky gut?

No, food sensitivities caused by leaky gut often improve as the gut lining heals. Once the intestinal barrier is repaired, your immune system is less likely to overreact to certain foods. However, it's important to reintroduce foods slowly and monitor your body's response.

12. Is leaky gut linked to weight gain?

Yes, leaky gut can contribute to weight gain by:
- **Increasing Inflammation**: Chronic inflammation can lead to insulin resistance and fat storage.
- **Disrupting Hormones**: Imbalances in gut hormones like ghrelin and leptin affect hunger and satiety signals.
- **Nutrient Deficiencies**: Poor absorption of nutrients can slow metabolism.

Healing your gut can improve weight management by reducing

inflammation and restoring proper hormone regulation.

13. Can children develop leaky gut?

Yes, children can develop leaky gut, especially if they have:
- Diets high in sugar and processed foods.
- Frequent antibiotic use.
- Food allergies or intolerances.
- Conditions like eczema or asthma, which are linked to gut health.

Encourage children to eat a diverse, whole-food diet and limit processed foods to support their gut health.

14. What tests can confirm leaky gut?

Diagnostic tests for leaky gut include:
- **Zonulin Test**: Measures levels of zonulin, a protein that regulates gut permeability.
- **Lactulose-Mannitol Test**: Assesses intestinal permeability by analyzing sugar absorption.
- **Comprehensive Stool Analysis**: Evaluates gut bacteria, inflammation markers, and digestive function.

Consult a healthcare provider to determine which tests are appropriate for you.

Conclusion

Embracing Lifelong Gut Health and Vibrant Well-Being

Healing your gut is not just a journey of addressing symptoms—it's a transformative process that reshapes your relationship with your body, mind, and overall health. As we've explored throughout this book, the gut is far more than a digestive organ; it's the command center for many critical systems, including immunity, mental health, hormone regulation, and energy production. By prioritizing gut health, you are laying the foundation for long-term wellness.

This conclusion brings together the core principles shared in the chapters, offering you a clear path forward for healing and maintaining a healthy gut for life.

1. The Power of Awareness

One of the greatest takeaways from this journey is the power of awareness. Recognizing the connection between your gut and the rest of your body is the first step toward healing. Your gut isn't isolated; it's intimately linked to your emotions, hormones, skin health, and even your cognitive function. By acknowledging these connections, you've already taken an empowered step toward transforming your health.

2. The Key Lessons from This Book

a. Healing Takes Time and Consistency

Gut health is not a quick fix; it requires patience and commitment. Whether you're repairing a leaky gut or maintaining long-term wellness, the strategies shared in this book—such as dietary changes, stress management, and supplementation—are most effective when applied consistently.

b. Food Is Medicine

The food you eat directly influences your gut health. A diet rich in prebiotic and probiotic foods, anti-inflammatory ingredients, and gut-healing nutrients is your strongest ally in supporting the gut lining and fostering a healthy microbiome.

c. Lifestyle Matters

Your daily habits—how you manage stress, sleep, move your body, and even how you eat—are just as important as what you eat. Incorporating mindfulness practices, regular exercise, and sufficient sleep creates an environment where your gut and body can thrive.

d. Your Gut Is Unique

Healing and maintaining gut health is not a one-size-fits-all process. Each person's journey is shaped by their unique symptoms, triggers, and goals. This book has provided tools to help you identify and address your individual needs, empowering you to make informed decisions about your health.

3. The Long-Term Benefits of Gut Health

Investing in your gut health isn't just about alleviating symptoms; it's about creating a ripple effect that improves your overall quality of life. As your gut heals and functions optimally, you may experience:

- **Better digestion**: Relief from bloating, irregularity, and food sensitivities.
- **Increased energy**: Improved nutrient absorption and reduced inflammation.
- **Balanced hormones**: Regulation of menstrual cycles, mood stability, and reduced PMS symptoms.
- **Clearer skin**: A glowing complexion free of acne, eczema, or rosacea.
- **Improved mental clarity and mood**: Less brain fog, anxiety, and depression.

- **Stronger immunity**: Fewer illnesses and better resilience to stress.

These benefits extend beyond the physical—they allow you to show up as the best version of yourself in all areas of your life.

4. Moving Forward: Your Gut Health Game Plan

Step 1: Implement What You've Learned

Take small, actionable steps each day to incorporate the strategies outlined in this book. Whether it's preparing a gut-healing meal, practicing mindful breathing, or adding a probiotic to your routine, every choice matters.

Step 2: Stay Curious

Gut health is an evolving field of research. Stay curious and continue to educate yourself about new developments in gut health science. Knowledge empowers you to make better decisions for your body.

Step 3: Listen to Your Body

Your body has a remarkable ability to communicate its needs. Pay attention to how you feel after meals, during stressful periods, or when you change your routine. Use these signals to guide your choices and adjust your approach as needed.

Step 4: Commit to Maintenance

Healing your gut is just the beginning. Maintaining a healthy gut requires ongoing care, but the effort is worth the lasting benefits. Make gut health a lifelong priority to enjoy vibrant health and vitality.

5. You Are Not Alone

One of the most encouraging aspects of this journey is the shared experience of others who have walked this path. Whether it's the inspiring success stories in this book or people in your own life, know that you're not alone. Community, support, and shared knowledge are invaluable tools as you continue your journey.

References

Below is a curated list of references and resources that support the information and strategies outlined in this book. These references include scientific studies, expert articles, and foundational texts on gut health, nutrition, and women's wellness. They provide additional context and validation for the topics discussed.

Scientific Journals and Research Articles
1. Fasano, A. (2012). Leaky gut and autoimmune diseases. *Clinical Reviews in Allergy & Immunology, 42*(1), 71–78. https://doi.org/10.1007/s12016-011-8291-x
2. Peterson, C. T., Sharma, V., Elmen, L., & Peterson, S. N. (2015). Immune homeostasis, dysbiosis, and therapeutic modulation of the gut microbiota. *Clinical and Experimental Immunology, 179*(3), 363–377. https://doi.org/10.1111/cei.12474
3. Bischoff, S. C., & Barbara, G. (2014). Intestinal permeability—a new target for disease prevention and therapy. *BMC Gastroenterology, 14*, 189. https://doi.org/10.1186/s12876-014-0189-7
4. Turnbaugh, P. J., Ley, R. E., Hamady, M., Fraser-Liggett, C. M., Knight, R., & Gordon, J. I. (2007). The human microbiome project. *Nature, 449*(7164), 804–810. https://doi.org/10.1038/nature06244
5. Mayer, E. A., Tillisch, K., & Gupta, A. (2015). Gut/brain axis

and the microbiota. *Journal of Clinical Investigation, 125*(3), 926–938. https://doi.org/10.1172/JCI76304

Books and Foundational Texts

6. Perlmutter, D. (2013). *Grain Brain: The Surprising Truth about Wheat, Carbs, and Sugar – Your Brain's Silent Killers*. Little, Brown Spark.
7. Chutkan, R. (2015). *The Microbiome Solution: A Radical New Way to Heal Your Body from the Inside Out*. Avery.
8. Axe, J. (2016). *Eat Dirt: Why Leaky Gut May Be the Root Cause of Your Health Problems and 5 Surprising Steps to Cure It*. Harper Wave.
9. Bland, J. (2014). *The Disease Delusion: Conquering the Causes of Chronic Illness for a Healthier, Longer, and Happier Life*. Harper Wave.
10. Mosley, M., & Spencer, C. (2015). *The Clever Gut Diet: How to Revolutionize Your Body from the Inside Out*. Atria Books.

Web Resources and Articles

11. National Institutes of Health (NIH): Gut microbiota research and its impact on health. https://www.nih.gov
12. Harvard Health Publishing. (2018). The gut-brain connection. https://www.health.harvard.edu/diseases-and-conditions/the-gut-brain-connection
13. Cleveland Clinic. (2021). Leaky gut syndrome: What is it, and what does it mean for you? https://my.clevelandclinic.org
14. Mayo Clinic. (2021). Probiotics and prebiotics: What you need to know. https://www.mayoclinic.org
15. Environmental Working Group (EWG). (2023). Guide to clean eating and reducing exposure to toxins. https://www.ewg.org

Scientific Reviews on Gut and Hormonal Health

16. Koren, O., & Goodrich, J. K. (2016). The influence of the gut microbiota on endocrine-related diseases. *Nature Reviews Endocrinology, 12*(6), 379–390. https://doi.org/10.1038/nrendo.2016.20
17. Clarke, G., Grenham, S., Scully, P., Fitzgerald, P., Moloney, R. D., Shanahan, F., ... & Cryan, J. F. (2013). The microbiome-gut-brain axis during early life regulates the hippocampal serotonergic system in a sex-dependent manner. *Molecular*

Psychiatry, 18(6), 666–673. https://doi.org/10.1038/mp.2012.77

Dietary and Nutritional Research

18. DeMeo, M. T., Mutlu, E. A., Keshavarzian, A., & Tobin, M. C. (2002). Intestinal permeability defect in irritable bowel syndrome: A pilot study. *Neurogastroenterology & Motility, 14*(6), 669–675. https://doi.org/10.1046/j.1365-2982.2002.00398.x

19. Wells, J. M., Brummer, R. J., Derrien, M., MacDonald, T. T., Troost, F., Cani, P. D., ... & Mercenier, A. (2017). Homeostasis of the gut barrier and potential biomarkers. *American Journal of Physiology-Gastrointestinal and Liver Physiology, 312*(3), G171–G193. https://doi.org/10.1152/ajpgi.00048.2015

20. Gibson, G. R., & Hutkins, R. (2016). The concept of prebiotics and their role in health. *Nature Reviews Gastroenterology & Hepatology, 13*(8), 491–502. https://doi.org/10.1038/nrgastro.2016.81

About the Author

Dr. Amelia Grace Harper is a leading expert in integrative health and functional medicine, specializing in gut health, hormonal balance, and women's wellness. With over 15 years of experience as a physician and wellness coach, she has dedicated her career to helping women transform their health through evidence-based, holistic approaches.

Dr. Harper earned her Doctorate of Medicine (MD) from the University of California, San Francisco (UCSF), where she focused on internal medicine and nutrition science. She later pursued advanced training in functional medicine, becoming a sought-after speaker and educator on topics like gut-brain health, autoimmune recovery, and the role of nutrition in hormonal harmony.

A passionate advocate for empowering women, Dr. Harper has worked with thousands of patients to uncover the root causes of their chronic health issues, including leaky gut, PCOS, and thyroid imbalances. Her compassionate, practical strategies blend cutting-edge research with lifestyle-focused solutions, making optimal health achievable for all.

In addition to her clinical work, Dr. Harper is a prolific writer, podcaster, and workshop facilitator. Her approachable style and relatable insights have earned her a devoted following in the wellness community. When she's not helping others unlock their health potential, Dr. Harper enjoys hiking in the mountains, experimenting with gut-friendly recipes, and spending time with her husband and two children in Boulder,

Colorado.

This book, *Healing from the Inside Out: Women's Guide to Overcoming Leaky Gut and Reclaiming Health*, is her latest contribution to empowering women to achieve lasting vitality.

Disclaimer:

The information presented in this book is for educational and informational purposes only and is not intended as professional advice. The author and publisher have made every effort to ensure the accuracy of the information; however, they assume no responsibility for errors, omissions, or any outcomes resulting from the application of the contents. Readers are encouraged to consult with a qualified professional for specific advice tailored to their situation.

All opinions expressed are those of the author and do not reflect the views of any affiliated organizations. The reader assumes all risks for the use of the material provided in this book. The author and publisher disclaim any liability for direct or indirect consequences arising from the use or interpretation of the information.

All rights reserved. No part of this book may be reproduced, distributed, or transmitted in any form without prior written permission from the author or publisher, except in the case of brief quotations used in reviews.

Copyright
© 2024 by Dr. Amelia Grace Harper
All rights reserved.

No part of this book may be reproduced, distributed, or transmitted in any form or by any means, including photocopying, recording, or other electronic or mechanical methods, without the prior written permission of the publisher, except in the case of brief quotations embodied in critical reviews and certain other noncommercial uses permitted by copyright law.

This book is a work of fiction/nonfiction. Names, characters, places, and incidents are products of the author's imagination or used fictitiously. Any resemblance to actual events, locales, or persons, living or dead, is purely coincidental.

First Edition: December, 2024

Printed in the United States of America

Legal Notice

This book is for informational and educational purposes only. While the author and publisher have made every effort to provide accurate and up-to-date information, they assume no responsibility for any errors, inaccuracies, or omissions. Any reliance placed on the information in this book is strictly at the reader's discretion and risk.

The content is not intended to replace professional advice, including but not limited to medical, legal, financial, or other professional services. Readers should consult with an appropriate professional for specific guidance related to their unique circumstances.

All trademarks, product names, and company names mentioned herein are the property of their respective owners. Their inclusion does not imply endorsement, affiliation, or sponsorship. Unauthorized reproduction, distribution, or transmission of this publication in any form is prohibited without prior written consent from the author or publisher.

By reading this book, you agree to indemnify and hold harmless the author, publisher, and any affiliated parties from and against all claims, liabilities, losses, or damages resulting from your use of the information provided.

Acknowledgments

This book would not have been possible without the support, guidance, and encouragement of many incredible individuals.

First and foremost, I want to express my heartfelt gratitude to my family. Your unwavering support, patience, and love have been my foundation throughout this journey. To my partner, thank you for believing in my vision and encouraging me to persevere, even during the most challenging moments. To my children, your curiosity and zest for life inspire me daily.

To the countless women who have shared their stories, struggles, and successes with me—you are the reason this book exists. Your resilience and determination to reclaim your health have been a source of profound inspiration. This book is dedicated to empowering more women to embark on similar transformative journeys.

I am deeply grateful to my mentors and colleagues in the fields of functional medicine, nutrition, and women's health. Your insights, research, and dedication to advancing the understanding of gut health have enriched this book and made it possible to share evidence-based, practical solutions with readers.

A special thanks to my editor, who turned my ideas into a cohesive and accessible narrative. Your expertise and attention to detail brought this book to life. To the publishing team, thank you for your professionalism and guidance in bringing this work to readers around the world.

Lastly, to you, the reader: Thank you for trusting me to guide you on your journey to better health. Your decision to prioritize your well-being is both courageous and inspiring. I hope this book provides the tools, knowledge, and encouragement you need to transform your health and live a vibrant, fulfilling life.

With deepest gratitude,

Dr. Amelia Grace Harper

www.ingramcontent.com/pod-product-compliance
Lightning Source LLC
Chambersburg PA
CBHW052248220526
45471CB00001B/236